DON'T EAT THAT!

INTERMITTENT
FASTING FOR LIFE

WE ARE WHAT
WE DON'T EAT

KHAREN MINASIAN

Table of Contents

DON'T
EAT
THAT!

Introduction

In India, long ago, there was a young prince who became disillu-sioned with his life at court and decided to leave the world and go off into the forest to pursue the life of an ascetic and mendicant. India actually has many such stories. Initially, his family was in shock. How could he leave his family and his privileged life of wealth, to go off and live like a beggar?

The prince's mother was a wise woman. She thought long and hard about her son's decision. Then she sent for her son and told him she had three pieces of advice for him, which were:

1. Always walk with family.
2. Always sleep in the most comfortable of beds.
3. Only eat the most delicious of foods.

The prince was understandably confused. He asked his mother, "How can I walk with family when I am leaving all of you behind?

And how can I possibly sleep in a comfortable bed, or eat delicious food when I have no money and no possessions?"

His mother answered him with a glimmer in her eye. "When you walk with another, it is that person who is now your family, for truly, we are all children of God. When you sleep, only do so when sleep overtakes you, and you will have the best and most comfortable sleep. And only eat when you truly yearn for food, so that no matter what you eat, it will taste like the most delicious banquet."

Her advice to 'only eat when you are truly hungry' is excellent advice for anyone, living in any age. We all know the feeling of hunger. But unfortunately, we don't experience this feeling often enough. We're fashioned by nature to experience hunger. It's programmed into our DNA; literally. Rather than warding off hunger through continual eating, we would be wise to embrace it. When we experience hunger, we should be pleased. It's our friend. Rather than fighting it off, we should be grateful, for at that moment, we are healing. Hunger informs us that we are strengthening and purifying our bodies, while we extend our lifespan.

Hunger, in this context, does not refer to starvation. Hunger is the craving your body expresses when your stomach is empty.

In the world today, everyone is continuously bombarded with messages about what we should eat. We can't avoid ads on TV, on the internet, within stores, magazines, newspapers, even billboards; entreating us to partake of this or that culinary pleasure. These ads for foods, and so-called foods, are ubiquitous. Our subconscious has become polluted with them. Is it any wonder that so many Americans are overweight?

According to the World Health Organization, worldwide obesity has tripled since 1975. In the United States today, 32% of the adult population, or about one in three, is overweight. But when you add to these overweight numbers, the 37% of American adults who are obese, now you have nearly 70%; seven out of ten adults, who are either overweight or obese. It's an epidemic.

But isn't obesity simply a matter of personal choice? If obese people are satisfied with their weight and the profile of their bodies, then why does their body composition matter? If they can accept the fact that they have three or four wardrobes in their closet and that they are tired and lethargic most of the time, then this is the life they have chosen for themselves, and we should not be concerned for them; right?

Obesity, in fact, has profound consequences beyond body image. It is a serious health and medical matter. It will shorten your life and sully the quality of the years you do have.

Obesity impacts the family of that person. They too have to endure the health consequences of their family member, including the depression that so often accompanies obesity. Obesity is a marker for a list of serious, potentially life-threatening chronic illnesses, like cardiovascular disease and diabetes. Obesity, and other components of metabolic syndrome, have also become recognized as correlative markers of Covid-19 patients who have to fight for survival.

Obesity is a problem for society at large, because, either directly or indirectly, it drives up health care costs. With it affecting 37% of the American adult population, it is in many ways a gravely serious issue.

Four or five million years ago, when the first human-like beings began to appear, earth life was very different. Prehistoric humans didn't have sprawling supermarkets to shop in or fast-food mongers on every other corner. They had to work and struggle for their sustenance. Establishing any kind of dietary regularity or consistency just wasn't feasible. The earliest humans did not farm. They had no stockpile of food. They foraged for herbs and hunted for game in real time.

Life was, quite literally, a process of continual feast and famine. After the kill of a small mammal or a few fish, prehistoric man would often go for days until he again found something to fill his belly with. Walking around for a few days without food was normal. For this ancient prehistoric being, the experience of hunger was an ongoing, unavoidable feature of life.

Evolution has a way of compensating for the everchanging environmental conditions that plants and animals face throughout their lifespans. But evolution takes time. Evolutionary response to environmental conditions is a slow process, normally taking many generations to develop.

What is important to recognize with respect to these ancient beings, is that our own physiology today is based upon the blueprint established by these prehistoric humans, ages ago. We have evolved with the ability to sustain life without food for short periods of time. Our bodies retain fats and nutrients, so that on days when we don't have ready access to food, we can survive off of our stored nutritional reserves.

These genetic patterns predate even our human ancestors. The life of a typical wild mammal is, and was no different. Food is eaten as it becomes available, or in the case of a predator, when it is killed. Lions, for example, routinely eat only every three or four days. They gorge themselves on a kill and then laze around for a few days until their bellies cry out for another.

So, these metabolic patterns are deeply ingrained, stemming from the very core of our genetic makeup, even predating the appearance of humanoids. Our bodies are designed to function optimally in feast and famine patterns. Nature has provided us with the means to accommodate this pattern, with our ability to store energy in fats.

The dilemma here is that now, we humans have so much food readily available to us, that our pattern has become feast and feast, without the famine in between. We don't give our body the opportunity to sustain itself off of our stored nutrients because we're constantly shoving more and more food into our mouths. Thank God we have sleep to create a daily fast. Sleep might be the only thing standing between us and mass suicide from eating.

"We are what we eat." This popular aphorism could not be more true. If you build a structure with the finest building materials available, your efforts will result in a well-built, durable building. Nutritious food is your friend and ally in your quest for a strong, healthy body and long lifespan.

"We are also what we don't eat." Too much of our modern diets involve foods that are not worthy to be called foods. We eat white, processed grains, refined sugars, pastas, and all manner of 'comfort foods' that the mind loves and the body hates. This destructive pattern of eating non-stop for sixteen hours per day, without a sufficient period of daily, or day-to-day fasting to help regulate caloric intake, compounded with the fact that the kinds of foods we do eat are even more likely to be stored as fat, has created a genetic/physiological conundrum.

Our physiological systems today do not reflect these fundamental changes in our eating/fasting patterns. In time, evolution should, at least theoretically, respond to these changing patterns. But this response will only manifest long after many future generations of people have come and gone. If only we could reason with our bodies; "Please stop storing so much fat. We have grocery stores now. We don't need to retain all of this anymore."

Evolution's slow response to environmental changes also manifests in other physiological processes. Our complex immune system, for example, is a marvelous evolutionary development that keeps us alive as a species with healing and protective safeguards. But now, humans, and the environments they live in, have transformed so drastically over the past few centuries, that the immune system now, all too often, responds to stimuli in ways that are inappropriate and even harmful to us. This discrepancy involves a class of modern pathologies known as autoimmune disorders.

This sluggish response to environmental changes necessitates that we humans take proactive steps to deliberately create patterns of living and eating that conform to our ancient genetic and physiological blueprint. This is where the value of intermittent fasting comes into play.

Intermittent fasting is the antidote to nature's lagging response to these changes. Intermittent fasting provides us with a mechanism to conform to what our bodies need and expect. Intermittent fasting elegantly mimics the optimal historic pattern of eating and fasting that the human body is actually designed for, and empowers us with a natural means to seek and maintain optimal healthspan and maximum lifespan.

It is for this reason that prolonged intermittent fasting is the most superior form of fasting for human beings to engage in.

Over the past several years, intermittent fasting has made its way into the limelight. There has been a significant media buzz over IF, with dozens of celebrities weighing in with their personal IF experiences. IF has now become more than a means to outsmart evolution. It is, for better or worse, society's latest darling 'fad' diet. According to google, intermittent fasting was the most searched dietary term in 2019.

Human beings love to play the role of sheep, looking to others for guidance in making decisions about nearly everything, especially diet. If you researched popular diets over the last fifty or sixty years, you would find over a hundred fad diets which have come and gone. Because this sudden popularity of IF is partly celebrity-driven, interest in it will ultimately wane.

However, this media buzz has produced a foothold for IF in human consciousness, especially the consciousness of health professionals. There is a growing body of scientific evidence that supports a myriad of health benefits of IF. The role of intermittent fasting in weight control and optimal health maintenance is here to stay. Yes, it's currently a dietary fad; but a fad with legs.

A percentage of the determined souls who choose to experiment with IF will realize its remarkable benefits and go on to incorporate it into their lifestyles. This includes integrative physicians who will utilize it more and more with other treatment modalities as a mechanism to support and enhance a variety of medical protocols.

Chapter 1

Transformational
FASTING

Before examining the practice and benefits of intermittent fasting, it is best to first view fasting from a broader perspective. Intermittent fasting, while being perhaps the most superior form of fasting for general application, is only one type of fasting, of which there are many. By also exploring these other approaches and methods, we can take away important information which may become applicable in developing our own personal intermittent fasting protocol.

Food has power. It has the power to sustain life and to help ensure the propagation of new life forms. It is a currency of political and economic power. Food is a medium of social intercourse, an ambassador between cultures. But perhaps food's greatest power may lie in our abstention from it.

Religions and nations have evolved out of fasts. Empires have toppled and alliances have formed. It is a tool of the greats; Jesus, Moses, Mohammed, Buddha, Gandhi. These men applied fasting to the transformation of societies and nations. They also incorporated it into their personal spiritual quests.

Fasting is a holistic medium of transformation. Anyone can utilize fasting for their own personal transformation: spiritual, psychological, emotional, and physical. Everyone fasts. We fast when we sleep. We fast between meals. We fast between snacks. Our bodies have evolved to utilize periods of fasting for repair and repose.

When we fast, our brain chemistry is altered. This alteration changes the way we think and feel. It alters mood, producing an anti-depressant effect, and a sense of well-being.

Fasting has been shown to relieve and successfully treat a number of medical conditions. Research conducted on human subjects has suggested that fasting is effective in improving hypertension, cardiovascular disease, diabetes, and cancer.

Fasting not only has the power to change our bodies for the better, it also has the power to transform our perceptions of the world and how we think. Fasting can induce altered states of consciousness, which can have significant therapeutic effects. Fasting can cause significant, meaningful personal insights and enhanced creativity. It has been known to completely alter a person's self-perception and worldview.

Fasting, as a spiritual discipline, is the most ancient form of asceticism, with examples found in nearly every religious and sacred tradition.

Modern medicine has discovered fasting to be a remarkable new therapy. As we fast, a robust set of self-healing mechanisms are launched. Many of these mechanisms are more active during fasting, than in any other state. Research suggests that these benefits are so far-reaching, as to cause certain medicines to work more effectively.

TYPES OF FASTS

Fasting is the voluntary abstention from food and/or drink over a specified period of time for health, spiritual, or political benefit. The most rigorous type of fast involves total abstention of all solid foods and liquids, including water.

There are many types of fasts. Fasts are often described by what a person does consume during the fast. In a water fast, the person consumes only water. In a juice fast, the person consumes fruit and vegetable juices, along with water. In a fruit fast, the person consumes fruits, water, and other juices. In a dry fast, the person consumes nothing; no solid food, liquids, nor water.

There is even now a chocolate fast, purported to support weight loss efforts. The chocolate fast is an example of yet another type of fasting, known as the mono-fast. The person consumes only one type of food for a specified period. The food is usually a fruit, such as grapes or watermelon. The mono-fast is also known as 'mono-diet', or 'mono-therapy'. Most health professionals consider the mono-fast to be a form of modified diet, and not a true fast.

Some fasts are described according to the fast's duration. A person may engage in a three-day, five-day, or fourteen-day fast. The duration of the fast may also be structured with consecutive on-and-off periods of eating and abstention. These fasts are known as intermittent fasts.

In medical terms, a fast is the metabolic state which is achieved once all previously eaten food is completely digested. This state can be achieved by eating the final meal of the day in the late afternoon or early evening, and then fasting throughout the night. Physicians often prescribe an overnight fast in preparation for serum draws, especially when testing for blood glucose, cholesterol, and lipids.

Therapeutic Fast – Water Only

A water-only fast, which is conducted and monitored under the supervision of a health professional, for the specified application as a medical intervention, is known medically as a therapeutic fast. A therapeutic fast is normally conducted in a near-complete state of rest. All non-essential activities are postponed until the fast is completed.

The International Association of Hygienic Physicians (IAHP) is a professional association of licensed, primary care physicians who specialize in therapeutic fasting. The IAHP has established a set of standards of practice.

1. Prior to initiating the fast, the physician collects a case history and performs a physical exam.
2. The physician consults with the patient regarding their medications, and any modifications to those medicines that are anticipated as being appropriate and necessary.
3. Serum monitoring of the patient, including appropriate lab tests, are conducted prior to the initiating the fast. Any fast beyond seven days requires continual physiological monitoring.
4. Physicians secure informed consent documents.
5. Vital signs to be monitored daily.
6. Physicians maintain a daily log of progress and vitals.
7. Water must be available to patients at all times.
8. Physician is responsible for post-fast monitoring, recuperation, and hygiene, until sufficient recovery is achieved.

A fast which is supervised by a qualified health professional limits the risks associated with water fasts, and increases the chances that the fast will have a successful outcome, physically and emotionally.

IAHP certified physicians, when monitoring a patient's fast, often look for certain markers, including:

1. How quickly is ketosis (fat burning) achieved
2. How quickly the patient leaves ketosis stage, after refeeding begins
3. The patient's quality of sleep during the fast
4. A rapid decrease in potassium levels
5. The presence of offensive odors (breath)
6. The presence or absence of hunger pangs
7. The presence of nausea and/or vomiting in the first few days of the fast
8. The possible presence of withdrawal symptoms

Clinics that provide therapeutic fasting services typically require patients to remain in the clinic during initial refeeding. Refeeding usually includes raw cooked vegetables and grains, along with fruits and fruit juices.

Dry Fasting

Dry fasting is sometimes referred to as an absolute fast or complete fast. It is the most extreme type of fasting. Dry fasting is significantly more difficult to do, and involves a higher degree of risk. Dry fasting is normally performed for shorter periods of time, perhaps a maximum of three days.

In the nineteenth century, an Austrian naturopath developed a medical protocol that included dry fasting as a treatment for a variety of illnesses. The treatment protocol was highly complex, involving periods of refeeding, and re-fasting. The program was essentially an early form of intermittent fasting. Various modified versions have since been developed over the decades, used primarily to facilitate detoxification.

In the mid-twentieth century, a Russian mystic named Ivanov, was in the habit of dry fasting for seven days at a time. He recommended that everyone perform a dry fast for forty-two hours each week. Ivanov's forty-two hour fast amounted to yet another early form of intermittent fasting.

A Russian doctor, named Filonov, has been using dry fasting with his patients for over twenty years. He calls his technique, the 'cascade method'. The cascade method begins with a day of dry fasting, followed by a day of eating. Then, the duration of each interval increases to two days fast, two days eat, and continues up to five days of each. This cascade method is a form of intermittent fasting.

Filonov recommends breaking a dry fast by drinking small amounts of water, very slowly. He suggests consuming two liters over a two-hour period. He then recommends soft foods, soups, juices, and water.

Filonov, in one of his books, claims to have successfully treated over forty medical conditions with dry fasting. His list includes:

- Migraine headaches
- Gastritis
- Infertility
- Parasites

- Viral and bacterial infections
- Irritable bowel syndrome
- Arthritis
- Hypertension

Filonov has concluded that dry fasting activates immune response and has anti-inflammatory benefits. He states that during a dry fast, the body destroys toxins in a process he describes as 'incineration', when the cell burns off toxic substances in a cellular process known as autophagy. Autophagy is the action of a damaged or diseased cell, self-destructing from enzymes which originate from within the same cell.

Filonov says that there are several contraindications for dry fasting, which include:

- Tuberculosis infection
- Cirrhosis of the liver
- Inflammation of the abdomen or respiratory system
- Heart arrhythmia
- Low body mass index
- Thrombosis
- Periods of pregnancy and lactation
- Early childhood, younger than 14
- Late adulthood, over 70

A health researcher, named Tonya Zavasta, recommends that anyone who is considering a dry fast, try it for 24 hours first, as a personal assessment. Zavasta dry fasts every day between the hours of 2:00 PM and 7:00 AM, which is again, a form of intermittent fasting.

Dry Fasts, Breatharians, and Death

The medically accepted period of time that a person can survive without water is three days. Dehydration sets in fairly quickly causing extreme thirst, fatigue, organ failure, and ultimately, death. The body needs water for nearly every physiological process. Without water, these processes cease to function.

For example, a reduction of water intake causes a drop in blood volume. With less blood circulating in the body, a severe drop in blood pressure will ensue, potentially leading to unconsciousness and/or death.

Three days is, however, a generalized benchmark, with the actual safe period for a particular individual being determined by:

- activity level
- overall health, including chronic conditions
- age, height, and weight
- gender
- climate, especially one's exposure to heat

Attempting to purify the body of toxins with dry fasting is counter-intuitive. Water, after all, is the medium used by the body to remove toxins from cells, and excrete them through urine. Without water, these toxins have the opportunity to build up. This toxicity harms the kidneys, whose job it is to remove toxins. If the kidneys fail, toxins build up further to dangerous levels.

A group of researchers, Marie Neeser, Patrick Ruedin, and Jean-Pierre Restellini documented the case of a prison hunger-striker who was admitted three times to the prison hospital, suffering from dehydration and acute kidney failure, after multiple extended dry fasting periods.

Dry fasting has been taken up by some spiritual leaders and seekers as a sadhana, or spiritual discipline. When incorporated into a spiritual context, dry fasting is known as 'inedia', or 'breatharianism'.

The claim behind dry fasting as a spiritual practice is that a human being can live directly off of prana, or life energy, without the need of food or water. We assimilate prana principally from the air we breathe; hence the name breatharian.

A self-proclaimed guru, named Ellen Greve, is an outspoken advocate of breatharianism. She calls it 'pranic nourishment'. Ms. Greve changed her name to 'Jasmuheen', to coincide with her guru persona. Jasmuheen has published several books on the subject.

Five deaths have been directly linked to Jasmuheen's teachings and publications. In one case, a 53-year-old Australian woman died in 1999 while attempting Jasmuheen's breatharian program. Two of Jasmuheen's followers were charged with manslaughter for their involvement in the woman's death. They were both convicted and served six-year and two-year prison sentences. Jasmuheen's response to the incident was that the dead woman was not coming from a place of integrity, and did not have the proper motivation.

A Scottish woman died, after attempting to survive solely on light, another of Jasmuheen's claims described in her writings. Another 22-year-old German man died the same way, attempting to live off of pure sunlight. A Dutch woman and a Swiss woman died under similar circumstances.

Juice Fasting

Juice fasting, as the name suggests, involves the consumption of juices and water only, over a specified period of time. Juice fasting can be scheduled as a prolonged fast, or as an intermittent fast. Prolonged juice fasts can be as long as fourteen days, or even longer.

There are various schools of thought as to how a juice fast should be conducted. For example, advocates of raw foods insist that a juice fast should only include pure organic raw juices, extracted from fresh fruits and vegetables. They insist that packaged and processed juices should be avoided due to their pasteurization. They further urge that juices should be consumed within thirty minutes of extraction and should not be refrigerated.

Juice fasting advocates believe that fresh, raw juices aid the body in expelling toxins associated with metabolism. They say that the body is actually incapable of processing and excreting these toxins under normal circumstances, and that juice fasting facilitates elimination.

Juice fasting is perhaps the most widely practiced form of fasting. It is performed at health facilities and retreats throughout the world. The Buchinger clinics in Germany define their protocol as follows:

"Buchinger's therapeutic fasting method is a modified fasting method. It supplies primarily carbohydrates (fruit juices and vegetable consumme) of approximately 250 kcal per day. These ingredients can be supplemented according to individual needs by proteins in the form of milk products, micro-nutritional elements (minerals, vitamins, micro-biotic foods)."

Rudolf Breuss, an Austrian naturopath, developed a 42-day juice fasting program, which he claims nourishes the body, while starving cancer. Breuss' juice blend included:

- Red beet root – 9.6 oz
- Carrots – 3.2 oz
- Celery root – 3.2 oz
- Small black radish – 1 oz
- One small potato

There appear to be some contraindications for certain people for juice fasting. This group is essentially the same population, contraindicated for water-only fasting. It includes:

- Young children
- Pregnant and lactating women
- People with liver and/or kidney problems
- People with low body weight and/or mass

Additionally, people suffering from certain chronic conditions, such as cancer, autoimmune disease, and certain other chronic diseases, should not juice-fast because the body needs more nutrients than usual, and a drop in nutritional intake could exacerbate their illnesses. People with diabetes should also consult with a health professional prior to juice fasting, since fruit sugars are quickly absorbed, making blood glucose levels rise too rapidly. This is also true with anyone diagnosed as prediabetic. Another factor is the lack of fiber in a juice fast. Fiber improves insulin sensitivity, helping to prevent or mitigate diabetes.

Many fasting experts suggest that water-only fasting is superior to juice fasting because water-only allows the body to rest, whereas juices require the digestion mechanisms to remain engaged. According to Naomi Neufeld, UCLA endocrinologist, water-only fasting allows for the following:

"Eventually the body burns up stored sugars, or glycogen, so less insulin is needed to help digest food. That gives the pancreas a rest. On juice diets, recommended by some spas, you may lose weight, but your digestive system doesn't get that same rest."

Green Juice Fast

Some fasting proponents believe that it is important to draw a distinction between a fruit juice fast, and a green juice fast. Green juice fasts, as the name implies, employ the juices of green vegetables, such as spinach, lettuce, kale, bell peppers, and celery. These green juices contain either no sugars, or only trace amounts of sugars, compared to fruit juices. Since leafy vegetables contain little actual juice, water is often added. Some advocates of green juice fasting grind up the dried, vegetable material, which is left over after juicing. They then add the powder to the green juice. This added powder provides nutrients and fiber. However, the solids do require the body's digestion process to engage.

Master Cleanse

The master cleanse is a type of juice fast, which is intended to detoxify the body, along with weight loss. It was developed by Stanley Burroughs in the 1940's. Like a juice fast, or water fast, it excludes all solid food.

The master cleanse has three components.

1. Upon awakening, the person fasting drinks a quart of water, to which is added two teaspoons of salt. An alternative to the salt water is one cup of herbal laxative tea.
2. Six to twelve glasses of lemonade are consumed throughout the day. Burroughs recommends purified or spring water, fresh squeezed lemon juice, organic maple syrup, and cayenne pepper.
3. In the evening, one cup of herbal tea is consumed.

The recommended duration of the fast is ten days. Some popular weight loss programs have adopted a shorter, modified version of the master cleanse.

Another health practitioner, Austrian physician Franz Mayr, developed a somewhat similar detox cleanse in the early 1900's, and is still used today by a number of European health clinics and spas. Mayr Therapy is a form of intermittent fasting administered over a period of one to three weeks. A combination of herbal tea with honey and lemon juice is consumed on fasting days. On refeeding days, the person consumes dry, white bread and milk. Mayr Therapy is often accompanied by breathing exercises and abdominal massages.

Another fasting proponent, Arnold Ehret, simplified the Mayr approach. He gave his fasters lemon juice, with a trace of honey and brown sugar. He claimed the mixture broke up mucus in the body.

There is no hard science that supports the detox effects of the master cleanse approach. Some researchers warn against a prolonged master cleanse fast, one exceeding thirty days. They cite the potential development of a deficiency of essential nutrients, such as vitamins, minerals, and proteins. However, some dietary weight loss systems, such as Medifast, have successfully incorporated versions of the master cleanse into their programs.

Another type of master cleanse involves the consumption of powdered functional foods, mixed with pure water or juice. These powders may include pure whey, body building formulae, and superfoods like spirulina, wheat grass powder, or barley powder. Practitioners often adopt these diets over prolonged periods. Most fasting experts consider the functional food approach a fad diet, and not a true fast.

Water fasting purists argue that any fast that includes anything other than pure water is not a true fast. The body does not get the same respite from glucose as it does with a water-only fast. Also, the process of ketosis, or fat burning, is retarded when solid nutrients are introduced into the fasting protocol.

Modified Fasts

Modified fasts are really strictly controlled diets that are designed to mimic the weight loss and detox effects of a water or juice fast. One of these approaches is called the "fat fast". Pure, healthy fats, like cream and butter, and vegetable oils, like coconut oil and olive oil, are allowed during the fast.

Eating fats in isolation by themselves in this manner, is not something we normally do. However, proponents of the fat fast claim that it makes the fast much easier, by curbing hunger urges, without lessening the physiological benefits of the fast.

They further claim that there are inherent benefits to adding these pure fats. The fats do not interfere with ketosis, and provide the faster with an energy boost and improved mental clarity. While there is no research to support these claims, there is a growing volume of anecdotal accounts which support the idea.

Chapter 2

Intermittent
FASTING

Intermittent fasting, or IF, is a method of fasting which has grown significantly in popularity in recent years. It is utilized primarily as a weight-loss system. But the benefits of IF go well beyond weight loss. The health and medical benefits of IF have been well-researched and documented.

IF involves a pattern of repeated fasting and refeeding, alternating between periods of fasting and non-fasting. The fasting periods can be dry, water-only, juice, or some other chosen form of modified fasting.

There are many ways to structure an IF program. There is no particular formula that appears to be superior to others. A person embarking on an IF program can experiment with various methods, to discover what seems to be easiest and most beneficial for them.

Research into IF originally began in the 1940's with animal studies. A 1945 study using rats concluded that the lifespan of rats who were placed into an IF program was significantly increased, compared to the control population. The control group received the same food every day. The test group was fed the same food as the control group, but fasted intermittently throughout the study. The IF group showed a 20% increase in lifespan for the males and a 15% increase for females.

Since these early studies, a significant body of scientific research has been conducted, both animal and human. While the outcomes of these studies vary relative to the focus of each study, they all unanimously agree that there are significant health benefits which can result from IF.

The term, hormesis, refers to a favorable biological response resulting from low exposures to toxins and other sources of physiological stress. With respect to aging and longevity, a hormetic phenomenon is characterized as a beneficial response to a stress, such as fasting. Several studies have suggested that IF may function as a form of beneficial hormesis, resulting in increased lifespan.

Traditional hunter-gatherer societies did not develop modern maladies, such as obesity and type II diabetes, even during periods when food was plentiful. With the agricultural revolution came an abundance and reliability of foodstuffs, and humans began the habit of eating two or three times each day. But these early diets were carbohydrate and meat-based, and did not lead to health problems like obesity. Obesity is modern-day health issue.

The primary factor here is our insulin response to food, since obesity is largely a problem associated with excessive insulin. With respect to insulin levels, the timing and frequency of eating appears to be as important as the composition of the meal itself. In other words, the question of when and how we eat is as important as what we eat.

The term 'intermittent fasting', refers to a dietary routine where periods of fasting occur regularly between periods of normal eating. How long each period lasts can vary significantly. There is no superior way to structure these two periods. One method may work best for one person, while another approach will work best for someone else. One person may prefer shorter fasts, while another person may prefer longer periods of fasting. It is essentially a matter of personal preference.

Fasting periods can range from twelve hours to several days. A person can do IF once per week, once a month, or once a year. Shorter duration fasts of less than twenty-four hours, are usually done more frequently, often daily. Longer IF durations, of one to two days, may be done once or twice per week.

Generally speaking, those who engage in IF for weight loss, tend to use shorter fasting periods of less than twenty-four hours. People who engage in IF for more serious medical issues, such as fatty liver disease, type II diabetes, or other metabolic disorders, will incorporate longer periods of fasting, such as one to seven days. Shorter fasting periods are much easier to do and do not involve nutritional deficiency risks. Shorter fasts also work best in conjunction with modern active lifestyles.

One proponent of IF, Certified Nutritionist Amy Berger, states:

"I think intermittent fasting is great. Done on a regular basis, the body gets accustomed to it and you don't think twice about it. Your hunger signals will become more regular – that is, they'll adjust to the fasting and you'll start to become hungry when your body is ready to eat, rather than from 'false' signals being driven by wild fluctuations in insulin, blood glucose, and stress hormones."

Once you begin on an IF program, you can always change your protocol. You're not locked into any one approach. The first few fasting periods will be difficult, with the body craving food, largely from habit. However, once these first few days are completed, like everything else in life, fasting becomes easier with experience.

The Traditional 12-Hour Fast

In previous years, especially prior to the 1970's, an intermittent fasting regimen of equal twelve-hour periods of eating and fasting was considered a normal eating pattern. A person would eat three daily meals, perhaps beginning with breakfast at 7:00 AM, and an evening meal at 7:00 PM. Then the following morning, you would break your fast with breakfast.

Two major changes to the standard 12-hour-on, 12-hour-off eating routine occurred in the 1970's. The first change was the publication of the USDA's 1977 "Dietary Guidelines for Americans" that year. Also known as the 'food pyramid', the revised 1977 guidelines changed to a high carbohydrate diet, with reduced fats. Diets which are high in carbohydrates, especially refined carbs, result in high levels of insulin, which cause people to gain weight, and eventually, to develop obesity.

The other change that began to occur in the 1970's was a gradual increase in meal frequency. In 1977, the average number of meals consumed by Americans was three per day; breakfast, lunch, and dinner. Over time, the meal frequency of Americans has increased. By 2003, the number of meals consumed had increased to nearly six per day, with the standard three meals, plus two or three daily snacks.

This evolution has resulted in a number of health issues and problems. When a person consumes just three meal per day, once each meal's digestion is completed, it still allows for some time, perhaps an hour or two, for fat-burning to take place. However, when snacks are consumed between meals, and after the final dinner meal, the body is not allowed sufficient time for any fat burning. Insulin levels, in this pattern, are maintained throughout the day at high levels, perpetually.

Over time, these high insulin levels can lead to insulin resistance, which exacerbates the high insulin levels. This, in turn, leads to obesity and prediabetes.

Daily 12-hour fasting periods, combined with a two or three meal pattern, allow the body to return to low insulin levels during the day. This in turn helps prevent insulin resistance and the development of obesity.

In the 1950's and 1960's, Americans ate more whole foods, with lower carbohydrate levels, and less refined sugars. The daily 12-hour fast was enough to prevent obesity. Obesity, in the 50's and 60's was comparatively rare. Today, in the United States, it is an epidemic, with 37% of Americans being obese. But while a 12-hour fasting routine may prove to be an excellent preventive measure, it is most likely not sufficient to reverse weight gain. Longer periods of fasting are needed for meaningful weight loss.

The 16-Hour Fast

The 16-hour fast is an intermittent fasting schedule that alternates an 8-hour period of feeding with a 16-hour period of fasting. For example, the first meal of the day, breakfast, might be consumed at 9:00 AM. The final meal, dinner, would be consumed no later than 5:00 PM. The fast, in this example, begins at 5:00 PM and continues throughout the night until the 9:00 AM breakfast.

So, in a 16-hour fast, the feeding window is eight hours. Some people choose to skip the breakfast meal, and only eat two meals. But regardless of how many meals are consumed, the eating window is eight hours.

The 16-hour fast is superior to the 12-hour fast, because you have an additional four hours per day of fat-burning. Since you sleep through half of the fast, it is not difficult to conform to the routine.

The 16-hour fast is a schedule that a person can easily adopt as a standard eating routine, and maintain throughout one's entire life, if desired. There are no health risks or contraindications associated with the 16-hour fast. The effects are all positive.

The LeanGains Method

A Swedish bodybuilder, Martin Berkhan, was an early proponent of the 16-hour fast, which he called the LeanGains method. Then, some years later, a book was published on the 16-hour fast, called "The 8-Hour Diet". The 16-hour fast is best combined with a low carbohydrate diet. Weight loss on this plan tends to be slow. But by adhering to it over time, you will find a steady loss in body weight.

The LeanGains method was developed with bodybuilders and fitness enthusiasts in mind. It is specifically focused on weight loss and lean muscle development. No calories are consumed during the fasting period, including calories derived from juices. However, non-caloric liquids, such as pure water, diet sodas, calorie-free sweeteners, black coffee, and tea, including herbal teas, are allowed.

The LeanGains method allows the person to choose the feed/fast time windows, but recommends establishing a set routine, and then consistently sticking with it. It is also recommended that feeding not take place right before a strenuous workout. For working people, Berkhan also recommends not consuming the major portion of your day's food while working. This particular recommendation is contrary to what many other fasting experts would most likely recommend. However, Berkhan's focus was on maximizing fitness and bodybuilding goals, so that outlook was a major factor in how he formulated his program.

Regarding what food is recommended on LeanGains, Berkhan, of course, includes large servings of protein-rich foods, even on non-workout days. He recommends carbohydrates over fats on training days. However, if one of your major objectives is weight loss, then he recommends cutting down on the carbs. Regardless of objective, he recommends whole and unprocessed foods as a rule. He allows for 'cheat days', but only in strict moderation.

On the LeanGains diet, you will automatically eat less carbohydrates than you normally would. This should result in a significant burning of stored body fats.

The 20-Hour Fast

The 20-hour fast includes 4 hours of eating and 20 hours of fasting, daily. Ori Hofmekler is the author of "The Warrior Diet", a 20-hour fasting program. His diet incorporates a feed/fast schedule developed by him, and stresses that meal timing is just as important as what we eat. He named his version of the 20-hour fast, the Warrior Diet, from inspiration derived from ancient warrior societies, like the Spartans and Romans. These ancient warriors often ate only once per day.

The Warrior Diet recommends eating only during a four-hour window, during the evening hours, resulting in a 20-hour daily fasting period. He claims that the parasympathetic nervous system works best with a nightly eating routine, and that this helps the body remain calm and relaxed during digestion. He further claims that eating at night supports ketosis, or fat-burning, during daytime hours.

The Warrior Diet also spells out a specific order of what to eat during the four-hour feeding window. It begins with vegetables, followed by protein, and then fat. After eating these initial foods, if one is still hungry, then some carbohydrates can be added at the end.

However, in a 20-hour fasting regimen, the 4-hour eating window need not be just at night. In fact, it is probably ill-advised to schedule the eating period in the evening, due to the weight-gain risks associated with nighttime eating. Hofmekler's offers no science to back up his claims regarding nighttime eating. The four-hour eating period in a 20-hour fast could take place at any time during a person's waking hours, perhaps commencing in the early or mid-afternoon.

Hofmekler's Warrior Diet also emphasizes consuming only natural, unprocessed foods, combined with high-intensity interval training. Combining a daily 20-hour daily fast with this type of intense physical activity is a recipe for certain weight loss.

While more difficult to maintain, the 20-hour fast, like the 16-hour fast, is a routine which could easily be incorporated as an eating/fasting pattern on a long-term basis, perhaps for one's entire life. Since the body is receiving daily nourishment, one need only be concerned with consuming enough calories and nutritional components, relative to daily activity levels and specific nutritional needs. Otherwise, there is no significant health-related risk or contraindication associated with it.

The Warrior Diet does allow for some snacking during the fast, but the snacking is supposed to be limited to raw fruits and raw vegetables, a few small servings of protein, and drinking fresh, unprocessed juices. Hofmekler claims that the consumption of a few servings of protein allows a person to maximize the 'fight or flight' response of the nervous system.

However, fight or flight actually has more to do with adrenal response than it does with neurological response. He further claims that these small protein servings will activate alertness, while stimulating the fat-burning process and boosting energy.

If one is ready to take the challenge of adopting a daily, 20-hour fasting routine, it would probably be advisable to design a personal program, based on eating preferences and individual goals. While becoming familiar with Hofmekler's Warrior Diet may be a good starting point, his insistence on nighttime eating is probably ill-advised.

Circadian Rhythms and Eating Patterns

Circadian rhythms are repetitive biological patterns that are established as a part of our body's day-to-day physiological routines. These patterns can involve repetitive behaviors and the release of hormones. Circadian patterns are seen in nearly all mammals. Most of our hormones, including the stress hormone cortisol, and the parathyroid hormone, are secreted in a circadian rhythm. Circadian rhythms also help regulate the release of insulin, which affects weight gain. The hormone ghrelin, which affects our appetite, also functions within circadian patterns.

Nighttime Eating and Weight Gain

In Paleolithic times, humans did not farm. They were hunter-gatherers, who sought out and consumed their meals during daylight hours. After the sun went down each day, there was not sufficient light available to find and consume food.

As a result, humans have developed circadian rhythms which are determined largely by available natural light, relative to season, and time of day. Some mammals, who are more nocturnal in nature, have developed circadian rhythms that are not influenced as much by sunlight. But early humans were not nocturnal in nature.

Since these hormonal circadian patterns are daylight-specific, it would seem logical that it may be more advantageous for us to eat during the day, while avoiding eating at night. In this regard, the science appears to support this notion.

A 2013 study used a group of overweight women to determine whether or not time-of-day eating patterns influenced weight loss/gain. The women were divided into two groups. One group ate their largest meal of the day at breakfast, while the other group ate the largest meal of the day in the evening. Both groups were fed the same 1400-calorie daily diet. The only difference between the two groups was when they consumed their largest meal.

The results of the study showed that the breakfast group lost significantly more weight than the dinner group. They lost more weight because the dinner group had a much higher rise in insulin after the meal than the breakfast group.

Another earlier 1992 study had essentially the same results, with evening insulin response being between 25% to 50% greater than morning insulin secretions. Since weight gain is largely driven by insulin, the higher evening insulin response resulted in more weight retention compared to the breakfast group.

There is also a widely recognized correlation between people who work night shifts, and obesity. Night shift workers tend to eat most of their food at night. This correlation is most likely also exacerbated by an increase in the stress hormone, cortisol, resulting from a disturbed sleep pattern, also regulated by circadian rhythm.

The University of Barcelona Study

A study of eating schedule habits, recently completed at the University of Barcelona, and published in the scientific journal, "Nutrients", gave new meaning to the term, 'biological clock'; the body's innate, circadian mechanism that understands that daytime is the proper time to metabolize calories, and that nighttime is when we fast. The study's authors also coined a new term: *eating jet lag*.

The study monitored eating schedules, specifically the eating schedules that people have during weekdays, compared to their weekend eating schedule. Since our activity routines during the week are oftentimes quite different from our routines on the weekend, our eating schedules often differ significantly.

This is especially true in Southern Europe, where young people quite commonly begin their evening meal on the weekends as late as 10 PM. Friends often gather for drinks in a club or bar in the early evening hours and then ultimately migrate to a nearby restaurant. These cultural patterns made Barcelona an ideal locale for such a study.

Eleven hundred and six young people, between the ages of eighteen and twenty-five, participated in the study over a two-year period. Researchers asked each subject to maintain a log in which they entered the start time-of-day of each of their three daily meals. Since the population of subjects was large, and the study's duration was long, the results and conclusions reported by the authors are considered to be highly valid.

Once all of the data was collected, the researchers created a daily midpoint, time-wise, for each day's three meals. These mid-points were separated into weekday midpoints and weekend midpoints. These midpoints often differed by as much as three and a half hours. In other words, a person who ate breakfast at 7:30 AM and dinner at 6:30 PM during the week, might eat breakfast at 11:00 AM and dinner at 10:00 PM on the weekends. This irregularity in eating schedules was referred to by the authors as 'eating jet lag'.

María Fernanda Zerón Rugerio, one of the principal authors of the study, commented on the results, saying;

> *"Our results show changing the timing of the three meals during the weekend is linked to obesity. The highest impact on the BMI (Body Mass Index) could occur when there is a 3.5-hour difference in eating schedules. After this, the risk of obesity increased, since we saw individuals who showed a 3.5-hour eating jet lag increase their BMI by 1.3. kg/m2".*

She went on to conclude:

> *"As a result, when food intake takes place regularly, the circadian clock ensures that the body's metabolic pathways act to assimilate*

nutrients. However, when food is taken at an unusual hour, nutrients can act on the molecular machinery of peripheral clocks (outside the brain), altering the schedule and thus, modifying the body's metabolic functions."

The University of Pennsylvania Study

A similar study, conducted in 2017 by University of Pennsylvania researchers, also concluded that consuming meals later at night can cause weight gain and lead to obesity. The study demonstrated that timing eating patterns later in the day can increase weight, insulin levels, and cholesterol levels. It also impairs fat metabolism, hormonal markers related to cardiovascular disease, and contributes to various other health problems. The study is thought to be the first experimental evidence of the metabolic consequences of a pattern of delayed eating.

Kelly Allison, senior author of the study, commented on the study's findings saying;

"While lifestyle change is never easy, these findings suggest that eating earlier in the day may be worth the effort to help prevent these detrimental chronic health effects… We have an extensive knowledge of how overeating affects health and body weight, but now we have a better understanding of how our body processes foods at different times of day over a long period of time."

These late-eating studies all suggest that weight gain and weight retention are driven by insulin, as much as they are driven by caloric intake. We know that late eating patterns cause higher insulin secretions, translating into weight gain, and without some dietary intervention, will result in obesity.

Obesity is a condition that results largely from a hormonal imbalance, perhaps even more so than a caloric imbalance. Eating at night may have had some degree of survival advantage in ages past, allowing for fat to accumulate. However, in the twenty-first century, survival has more to do with losing fat than in accumulating and retaining fat.

Appetite and Hunger Rhythms

Hunger and appetite also have a circadian rhythm. When we awake in the morning, our hunger level is low. Breakfast is the smallest meal of the day, for most people. Low appetite in the morning is counter-intuitive, since we have just completed a fast of eight hours, or longer. Therefore, it would seem logical that the morning should be a time when we are the hungriest. If hunger is not simply a function of lack of food, then what is it that drives hunger?

Hunger is driven by a natural circadian rhythm, which is independent from our eating and fasting schedule. This circadian rhythm is caused by the hormone, ghrelin, commonly known as the hunger hormone. Ghrelin levels rise and fall during the day, with a low at around 8:00 AM, and a peak at around 8:00 PM. Our levels of hunger correlate with these two daily extremes.

Hunger patterns, therefore, are a function of our genetic and physiological make-up. It is not simply a matter of, "lack of food causes hunger". Hormonal patterns, to a large extent, determine when, and to what degree we are hungry. The conundrum here is that we experience our peak hunger levels at 8:00 PM at night. As we have just learned, from the results of numerous research studies, 8:00 PM is when we do not want to eat, if we are concerned about our weight and our metabolic health.

During prolonged fasts of three days or more, ghrelin levels peak during the first two days, and then drop off steadily. This pattern parallels hunger patterns during a prolonged fast. In a prolonged fast, hunger is a serious issue for the first 48 hours. After the first two days, hunger subsides.

Optimal IF Meal Timing

Any intermittent fasting program, regardless of the durations of the eating and fasting periods, should be designed with these hormonal circadian rhythms in mind. Whether the eating window is four hours, six hours, eight hours, or twelve, the most advantageous time of the day to eat our main meal is in the afternoon, between noon and 4:00 PM.

Why eat a big meal in the morning, when we have a suppressed appetite? It is almost like we're force-feeding ourselves. It's not a smart strategy. Eating later in the evening is likewise not a smart strategy. Eating large meals early and late will prove to be counterproductive to our weight loss efforts.

The so-called Mediterranean diet has gained wide popularity over the years, relative to nutritional content. But Southern Europeans also have a Mediterranean eating pattern. The largest meal of the day is normally lunch, which is often followed by a nap. Their breakfasts are modest, and dinner is often no more than a snack. The real value of the Mediterranean diet may be more associated with meal timing, than to nutritional considerations.

Chapter 3

Practical Approaches to Intermittent FASTING

In chapter 2, we explored the various IF protocols, including some specific programs designed by nutritional and fasting experts. Here in this chapter, we will explore some additional programs, also designed by researchers and experts. While some of the examples here will parallel what is presented in chapter 2, each program has some of its own unique elements, so as you will discover, they are not exactly the same.

Dr. John Berardi of Precision Nutrition

John Berardi is a nutrition and dietary expert who conducted his own personal research on intermittent fasting. He refers to himself as a professional dieter, having experimented with virtually every established dietary protocol in order to test its efficacy. With all of the recent interest in IF, he decided he would experiment with various methods to see what worked and to see if he could stick with them. It should also be added that Dr. Berardi is a seasoned track athlete and fitness expert.

He decided on six IF approaches to investigate. Of those six, he came away with three basic, practical methods that he feels combine effectiveness with a high probability of subject compliance. Dr. Berardi monitored his body weight, body fat percentage, blood and hormonal markers, and practical factors, such as energy levels and cognitive processes.

During the six-month testing period, Dr. Berardi watched his own body fat trim down from 10% to 4%, while his weight dropped from 190 pounds to 170 pounds.

Over his six-month testing period, he discovered two protocols that he could adhere to easily. He states that he was able to achieve the goals he had established at the outset in a way that was easier and less time-consuming than traditional dieting.

Two valuable points he discusses in his book are:

- A period of trial fasting is a valuable way to practice managing hunger, and an essential skill for anyone who wants to get in shape and lose weight.
- Fasting more regularly made it easier for him to achieve the benefits of IF compared to longer fasting periods and conventional diets.

Dr. Berardi's Favorite IF Protocols

Dr. Berardi's trial fast is 24-hour period, used to introduce the faster to the experience of hunger. Dr. Berardi incorporates late feeding into his dietary regimens. Late feeding is not recommended by many fasting and nutritional experts because scientific research has tied it to weight gain and risks for obesity. Since Dr. Berardi is a fitness enthusiast, he may have been introduced to the theory of late eating from the 'Leangains' method, developed by Martin Berkhan, also a fitness expert. Since Leangains recommends late eating, Dr. Berardi may have adopted the idea from Leangains. Another potential adaptation to Berardi's trial fast is to extend it to a 36-hour period, commencing on the last meal of day #1, and then breaking fast on the morning of day #3. It may also be advantageous to experience two trial periods, the first being 24 hours in duration, and the second, 36 hours in duration.

#1 - The Trial Fast

In the trial fast, you simply go without all food for 24 hours. The purpose is to experiment with the feeling of hunger, to get familiar with it, embrace it, realizing that feelings of hunger are natural and not harmful. Choose any 24-hour period that is convenient for you.

10 PM – Day 1

- Eat your final meal of the day
- Drink 16 oz of pure water

10 AM – Day 2

- Drink 1 quart of pure water with a serving of green superfood powder (spirulina, barley grass, wheat grass, etc.)
- Drink one cup of green tea
- Take 5 grams of protein powder (BCAA)

3 PM – Day 2

- Drink 1 quart of pure water with a serving of green superfood powder (spirulina, barley grass, wheat grass, etc.)
- Drink one cup of green tea
- Take 5 grams of protein powder (BCAA)

10 PM – Day 2

- Eat a small snack or meal
- Drink 16 oz of pure water

Day 3

- Eat normally

Dr. Berardi states that the powdered superfoods, green tea, and aminos are not absolutely necessary on the trial fast, but he includes them because he believes that they make the fast easier. They also provide some important micronutrients and an energy boost from the tea.

He says that drinking plenty of water during a fast helps to mitigate the hunger pangs. To overcome the boredom of drinking all that water, he adds a teaspoon of organic apple cider vinegar to each 8 oz of water.

During the trial fast, pay attention to your body. Are you stressed out or feeling upset? This is what hunger feels like. Experience it. Don't let hunger be a green light to snacking. The more you allow and embrace the feeling of hunger, the easier it is to manage. When you break your trial fast, do it with a snack or small meal of healthy food.

#2 - The Periodic Fast

The periodic fast switches back and forth from eating to fasting. The fasting period is normally a full day; either 24 hours or 36 hours long. Dr. Berardi recommends using the trial fast protocol for the fasting day.

He recommends choosing one day out of the week for the fast. Ideally, fasting days will be days that do not require a large amount of physical exertion. He recommends choosing a day where you are least likely to be stressed out. After developing the habit of fasting one day per week, he suggests that the faster may want to experiment with two days of fasting, to see how it goes.

In discussing the periodic fast, he softens up on the nighttime eating model, stating that the fasting period can also go from breakfast to breakfast. So, if your fast begins on the morning of day #1, you would break your fast on the morning of day #2 with a light breakfast.

This protocol of fasting one out of seven days has been popularized by some celebrities, including Coldplay's Chris Martin. He calls the protocol the 6:1 diet.

#3 - The Daily Fast - 16:8

Berardi's daily fast is his interpretation of the Leangains method of IF, with a strict daily eating period of eight hours, and a daily fasting period of sixteen hours. He states that after much experimentation, 16:8 has become his method of fasting.

He believes that the 16:8 method is best for people who already have good eating habits and are in reasonably good shape. He states:

- The 16:8 method will be more difficult for men who carry >15% body fat and women who carry >22% body fat.
- Men tend to find the 16:8 method easier than women.
- Women typically need a longer eating window, so he suggests trying 14:10, with a ten-hour feeding period.

Dr. Berardi does not cite any research or source for these opinions. Rather than adopt the arbitrary belief that the 16:8 method might be too difficult for someone to attempt, it is probably wiser to just go ahead and try the schedule to see how it goes for you. He recommends combining the 16:8 diet with:

- High protein foods
- Fresh vegetables
- Resistance training, three times per week, immediately prior to the day's first meal, which should be the day's biggest meal
- On the three training days, add a serving of carbohydrates

He states that the last meal of the day could come as late as 9 PM, which would place breakfast at 1 PM. However, it may be advantageous to shift these times earlier, perhaps eating the first meal at 10 AM and the final meal at 6 PM. Berardi's typical workout day on the 16:8 schedule looks like this:

8:00 AM

- Drink 16 oz of pure water

9:00 AM

- Drink a quart of water with a serving of green superfood powder, followed by a cup of green tea

11:00 AM

- Drink a cup of green tea

12:00 Noon

- Workout session with 10 grams of protein during workout

1:30 PM

- Eat first meal, and day's largest

4:30 PM

- Eat second, medium-sized meal

8:30 PM

- Eat final, medium-sized meal of day

Berardi claims that all of the components; resistance training, meal timing, and food selection are part of a strategic formula. If the feeding window is too tight, he recommends adding one or two hours and then eventually reducing down to eight hours. No matter what IF protocol someone chooses, he recommends always beginning with the trial fast.

More Fasting Protocols:

The 8-Hour Diet

This plan is a version of the 16:8 intermittent fast, devised and published by Men's Health Magazine editor, David Zinczenko. While similar to Berardi's approach, Zinczenko has devised his own set of protocols.

Bodhimaya Method

Bodhimaya Method is yet another 16:8 intermittent fasting protocol, developed by the award-winning luxury mind and body rejuvenation retreat company, Bodhimaya. This method has been popularized in recent years by various celebrities, like Kate Moss.

The Bodhimaya Method is an IF system, designed around the most current nutrition, anti-aging, and disease prevention science. They promote their system as a way to support the body's natural healing and repair processes, leading to younger looking skin, improved cognitive function, overall health benefits, and longevity. They view weight loss as a by-product of their program.

The Bodhimaya Method is a structured four-week program, that allows for each person to adjust their level of commitment to the program as they go. It begins with the simple task of eliminating between-meal snacks, and ends on an optional weekend of juices, smoothies, and soups. It also comes with recommended recipes and some fairly strict nutritional target guidelines.

Intermittent fasting is at the heart of the Bodhimaya program. They view fasting as an opportunity for the body to focus its attention on rejuvenation and repair. Therefore, the first principal is: 'no snacking'. No grazing allowed. They also stress the need to cut sugar intake down to a minimum.

Bodhimaya uses a standard 16:8 fast/feed schedule. The timing of the eight-hour window can be defined by the faster. It actually incorporates two 'golden ratios'. One is 16:8. The other is 1:7:2. This ratio informs the person what nutritional components are allowed each day: one portion of carbohydrates, seven portions of fresh fruit and vegetables, and two portions of protein. The experts at Bhodimaya have concluded that this is the magic nutritional ratio for maximum rejuvenation. They claim that the daily 16-hour fasting window, combined with their nutritional ratio, ensures that the body has everything it needs to repair itself.

The plan allows for the faster to cheat occasionally during the four-week period, especially on weekends. They want participants to have a relaxed, stress-free experience. They state that at 80%

of compliance, the faster will reap all, or nearly all of the targeted objectives. For heartier souls, they suggest the option of adding a one-weekend fast to the program, fasting from Friday evening to Monday morning. Bodhimaya takes a holistic approach to rejuvenation, recommending the incorporation of stress management techniques, such as meditation.

WEEK 1-

The objective during the first week is to prepare the body for longer daily fasting periods, by eliminating between-meal snacking. Their other week #1 recommendation is to begin to discipline food intake, by making positive nutritional choices. The first week, therefore, increases fasting periods between meals.

WEEK 2 –

The second week builds on week #1, by adopting the 1:7:2 nutritional ratio. They further recommend eliminating foods that have a negative nutritional impact, such as sugars, alcohol, caffeine, wheat, and dairy. They even recommend eliminating or cutting back high-sugar natural foods, such as dates, honey, maple syrup, and agave syrup. They also recommend sourcing carbohydrates from whole grains, such as brown rice, raw oats, and vegetables like sweet potato, or squash. There is no calorie counting with their method.

WEEK 3 –

On the third week, the program calls for strict adherence to the 16:8 IF fast/feed windows.

WEEK 4 –

During the fourth week, they recommend adding a prolonged, two-day semi-fast, beginning on the evening of day #1, and terminating on the morning of day #3. During this semi-fast, the only foods allowed are juices, smoothies, and soups. This semi-fast can take place during the fourth week or at the end of the fourth week.

ONGOING –

Bodhimaya states that their entire method can be incorporated into a person's ongoing lifestyle, becoming their standard, day-in, day-out fast/feed routine. They also recommend doing the three-day juice-smoothie-soup semi-fast every six months.

The Two Meal Day

The Two Meal Day fast is essentially the same program as the 16:8 fast. Developed by fasting maven, Max Lowery, the Two Meal Day protocol calls for skipping one of your meals on fasting days; either the first meal of the day or the last. What this does, in effect, is reduce the feed window down from twelve or fourteen hours, to eight. A person can select as many fasting days as he chooses, from one per week to all seven days per week.

You can even reduce the feed window down further, depending on when the faster eats his meals. For example, if you were to eat your first meal at noon, and then eat your evening meal at 6:00 PM, your fast is actually 18:6. Lowery does allow for a small snack between the two meals. His program calls for the feeding time window to remain undefined. He instead relies solely on sticking to two meals, regardless of when they are consumed. And unlike some of the modified IF 'diets', there is no need to calorie-count on dieting days.

He insists that the Two Meal Day program can be adopted over the long haul, even becoming a person's eating pattern for life. Lowery has been eating on the Two Meal Day plan since 2013. Unlike Berardi's daily 16:8 fast, Lowery does not prescribe any specific foods, or other components, like resistance training. He says to eat what you would normally eat, but just skip either your first daily meal or your last one. However, he does strongly recommend that along with the two-meal regimen, that fasters begin to develop better eating habits with nutritious natural foods.

Lowery says that by adopting the two-meal routine as a standard feeding plan, both body and mind have the opportunity to adapt to the program and establish it as a routine habit. He also states that once the glucose and fat-burning process kicks in, the faster can eat big, satisfying meals without interrupting it. He specifically doesn't want to tie the feed/fast windows to a specified time frame, because people tend to focus too much on the time of day, becoming obsessed with approaching eating times. He wants people to listen to their bodies and eat when real hunger sets in, rather than forcing ourselves to eat according to a rigid time schedule.

As far as a preference, whether to skip breakfast or dinner, he says it's a matter of personal choice. However, he adds that skipping breakfast has some good science behind it, with better biomarkers for insulin, cholesterol levels, and decreased body fat, compared to skipping dinner. He also feels that socially, it is probably easier for most people to skip breakfast.

The 5:2 Diet

Dr. Michael Mosley developed what he calls the 5:2 diet. This method combines five days of eating each week, with two days of restricted eating, limiting calories to 800/day. While not a true fasting protocol, it does accomplish many of the same things that a conventional IF method would accomplish. Researchers have been able to verify improved DNA repair and increased cognitive function, along with an increase in fat burning. As he was developing this program, Dr. Mosley experimented on himself. Over twelve weeks, he lost 20 pounds. He also had his blood sugar and cholesterol levels drop to normal after being prediabetic with high cholesterol.

The Blood Sugar Diet

Another semi-fasting protocol, developed by Dr. Michael Mosley, the Blood Sugar Diet has been formulated to prevent and help reverse type II diabetes. The program calls for eating three small meals daily, totaling no more than 800 calories, and continuing on the program for eight weeks.

The 1:1 Diet

This diet was developed by Dr. Krista Varady and Bill Gottlieb. It is patterned after the alternate day fasting regimen, with alternating days of feed and fast. The difference with the 1:1 diet is that, like the 5:2 method, it is not a true IF regimen. On the fasting days, the subject consumes 500 calories. You can eat what you would normally eat, but it has to be limited to 500 calories.

The Metabolic Balance System

Metabolic Balance is a simple program, devised by Dr. Wolf Funfack. The program merely calls for a strict 5-hour fasting time window between a person's three daily meals. So, if a person eats breakfast at 8:00 AM, lunch would be eaten at 1:00 PM, and dinner would be consumed at 6:00 PM, or later.

What this IF program achieves is it eliminates between-meal snacks. It also allows for enough time between feeding periods for the body's fasting metabolism to trigger glucose and fat-burning between meals. The Metabolic Balance approach has been adopted by many nutritional therapists around the world, and was widely publicized when Sam Smith and Kirstie Allsopp used it to trim their weights down.

Buchinger Wilhelmi –

Wilhelmi's program calls for longer periods of fasting, ranging from four days, up to twenty-one days. This program is actually a modified IF protocol, since it allows for small amounts of food, up to 250 calories, each day. They also recommend some carefully regulated exercise during fasting periods, to help retain muscle health and strength.

Chapter 4

Therapeutic Intermittent
FASTING

Alternate Day Fasting

Intermittent fasting routines that are structured with intraday feeding and fasting windows, like the 12-hour fast, or the 16-hour fast, are fairly simple to implement. They do involve some adjustment to our eating patterns. They also require some self-discipline to adopt, especially in the beginning stages. But over time, these daily feed/fast windows can be adopted as ongoing schedules, perhaps throughout our entire lives, since there are little or no health-related risks involved. Once new habits are established, compliance is fairly easy to maintain. The primary objective with these feed/fast schedules is usually weight loss.

Intermittent fasting protocols that are structured with longer durations of fasting; a day or longer, take a significantly more serious approach to fasting. These protocols are normally adopted for limited time durations, rather than adopting them as long-term habitual fast/

feed patterns. Intermittent fasting protocols that utilize longer periods of fasting are generally known as alternate day fasting, or ADF. ADF fasting programs are typically implemented for a week or a month, or perhaps for a number of months. Often, the objectives of ADF programs go beyond mere weight loss. An ADF program may be adopted in order to support some type of long-term physiological healing or transformation.

There are many ways to structure an alternate day fasting regimen. Fasting periods can be a single day, or multiple days. For example, a routine of two days of eating, followed by one day of fasting, is one way to structure an ADF regimen. The most common structure for an ADF regimen is one day of feeding followed by one day of fasting, repeated over a specified period. A one-day fasting window is actually a day and a half, or 36 hours, since the fasting period begins in the evening of the first day and continues until breakfast on the third day. For example, the last meal of the first day might be consumed at 7:00 PM. Two days later, at 7:00 AM, the fast is broken, resulting in a 36-hour fast.

Alternate Day Fasting and Prevention

Up to now, most of the research conducted on fasting, including intermittent fasting, has been done from the perspective of its ability to treat and heal existing health conditions, such as obesity and type II diabetes. The results of these studies demonstrate, unequivocally, fasting's curative and healing potential. But can fasting also be effective in providing preventive effects, to help protect us from disease?

A 2019 study, published in the medical journal, "Cell Metabolism", suggests that fasting does afford a variety of preventive qualities. The study, entitled *Alternate-day Fasting Improves Physiological and Molecular Markers of Aging in Healthy, Non-obese Humans*", is the first controlled trial, aimed at quantifying the effects of short-term ADF on a wide array of health markers, including physiological, biochemical, cardiovascular, and anthropometric, in a population of healthy adults.

One of the features of this study that strengthens its validity is that, along with the experimental and control groups, the study also included thirty participants who had been engaging in ADF for at least six months prior to the study's commencement. This allowed researchers to gain insight into the possible long-term benefits of intermittent fasting, by comparing experienced fasters to non-fasters.

In addition to the thirty experienced fasters, they selected sixty participants who were divided into two groups randomly. One of these groups was a group of new ADF fasters, and the other group was a control group who consumed their regular diet throughout the duration of the study. The four-week study included normal weight people, all between forty-eight and fifty-two years of age.

Those in the ADF group were instructed to eat and fast on alternate days. On their fasting days, no calories were allowed to be consumed. They even omitted dietary sodas. The only substances which they were allowed were water, carbonated water, unsweetened teas, and black coffee. On feeding days, there were no restrictions placed on them in terms of the amount or kind of foods consumed.

The comprehensive study measured physical markers, such as body weight, bone density, lean mass, fat mass, bone mass, bone mineral density, and total body composition. Researchers also measured serum samples for insulin, c-peptide, testosterone, cortisol, thyroid hormones, appetite hormones, oxidative stress markers, vitamin D, estrogen, and fatty acids. Many of these biochemical elements are associated with aging and longevity, hormone health, metabolic factors, and cardiovascular health. They also monitored blood pressure, heart rate, blood vessel elasticity, and markers associated with fat-burning.

Researchers monitored the level of compliance within the fasting group. They discovered that the group was nearly 100% compliant with their fast/feed routine of eating one day, and fasting the next day. They were compliant throughout the entire four-week testing period.

The fasting group reduced their average weekly caloric consumption by 37%. Coincidently, the control group, the group that ate their normal diet during the test's duration, also reduced their average caloric intake by 8%.

Their results for the ADF group showed the following results:

1. With respect to body composition, the ADF group had a significant reduction in Body Mass Index and fat mass.
2. Most of the fat loss was in the body's midsection, or belly fat. Belly fat is well-known to be the most toxic type of fat for a person to carry.
3. ADF improved the ratio between lean mass to fat mass.
4. Their cardiovascular measures were improved significantly. This included blood pressure and arterial stiffness.
5. Their risk for developing cardiovascular disease over the next ten years was lowered by 1.4%, which the researchers considered to be highly significant.
6. A thyroid hormone, known as fT3, was reduced. A reduction in fT3 is associated with increased lifespan in humans.
7. The levels of ketone, associated with fat burning, were elevated throughout the testing period, including feed days, which is when the blood draws were taken.

Researchers also compared data between the control, non-fasting group, and the experienced ADF fasters. The results of these comparisons showed the following results:

1. The long-term ADF group consumed a lower weekly caloric intake, eating 8700 calories per week, compared to 12,300 calories per week for the control, non-fasting group; a 28% difference.
2. The long-term ADF fasters had lower cholesterol levels.
3. They also had lower triglyceride levels.
4. They also had a lower resting heart rate.
5. They had lower levels of a pro-inflammatory marker, sICAM-1, which is associated with superior general health and longevity.

6. They had an increase of ketone bodies (BHB), which have been associated with increased lifespan and healthspan, improved metabolic health, and improved cognitive function.

All of the other measurements supported the fact that the long-term ADF group had no adverse effects from their >6 months of intermittent fasting.

The researchers also dug deeper, into molecular levels, looking at differences in genetic cycles. They discovered 54 metabolic-related genes which were all increased by at least 20%. This included pathways related to omega-3 and omega-6 fatty acids, and mitochondrial fat metabolism. Stress-response pathways and autophagy regulators were also significantly increased as well.

These results demonstrate that in just four weeks of intermittent fasting by healthy, fifty-year-old adults, a person's cardiovascular and metabolic health can be improved significantly. ADF is clearly an eating regimen that supports and enhances our evolutionary and circadian physiology.

The Alternate Day Diet

One of the leading proponents of alternate day fasts is Dr. James Johnson. Dr. Johnson calls his program the Alternate Day Diet. Dr. Johnson states that he learned over time in dealing with patients with weight-gain-retention and obesity problems, that it is nearly impossible for people to consistently maintain a caloric restriction discipline over the long haul while on a normal three-meal-a-day eating routine. In other words, sticking to a so-called 'diet', with the goal of long-term weight loss and weight management.

Dr. Johnson developed his Alternate Day Diet initially for his own use and benefit. However, he soon realized its great value in losing and maintaining healthy weight, and decided to develop it into a program for general use by everyone. He believes that his model is especially beneficial for people who already have good self-discipline, and who have a specific weight goal in mind.

Johnson's Alternate Day Diet, however, is really more like a traditional diet than it is an IF program. The routine is fairly simple. On one day, the dieter eats as he normally would. On alternating days, the dieter eats very little. Dr. Johnson recommends cutting caloric intake down to 20% of normal on dieting days. For example, if your normal caloric intake is 2000 calories per day, on alternating days, you would consume only 400 calories. Instead of dieting every day, you diet every other day.

The program does require a bit of inquiry into how many calories are appropriate for a normal eating day. Each person's daily caloric intake requirement varies widely, determined by several factors, such as age, gender, and activity level. There are several reliable sites on the internet which will assist a dieter in determining his own personal daily caloric requirement.

As a way to simplify the process of determining caloric intake on low-calorie days, Dr. Johnson suggests the dieter consider consuming meal replacement shakes, because they are developed and packaged with a standard, predetermined number of calories. He adds that he only recommends using the shakes in the beginning stages of the diet. Ultimately, he recommends eating normal food on each day of the diet, both feeding days, and low-calorie days.

The principle benefit of the Alternate Day Diet is reliable, sustained weight loss. Dieters typically report a loss in weight of at least one to two pounds per week. Another benefit to Johnson's approach is that there is no special food required. No change is needed with respect to one's normal choice of foods. He does, however, recommend eating unprocessed and whole foods. He also warns against binge eating on normal eating days. According to Dr. Johnson, binging on normal eating days poses the greatest risk with his program.

Since the dieter is eating every day, and only has to cut calories two or three days a week, it is fairly easily to comply with the program. It may be a bit difficult to initiate the new routine, but after establishing a new habit, compliance becomes easier.

The Alternate Day Diet is another IF-related dietary program that could be adopted over the long term, as long as a person's basic nutritional requirements are met.

The Eat Stop Eat Program

Eat Stop Eat is a traditional intermittent fasting model, developed by Brad Pilon. It is an especially good approach to IF for people who are already in the habit of eating healthy, nutritious food, but who want to drop weight rapidly.

In the Eat Stop Eat program, a one-day fast is completed once or twice weekly. During the fasting days, the person can drink calorie-free beverages, like coffee, teas, diet sodas, and pure water. You essentially take a break from normal eating for a day at a time, and then continue with your regular eating schedule after each one-day fast.

Pilon stresses the need to continue a normal eating routine, partly for psychological reasons. By not altering our normal dietary pattern, the body and mind are less likely to rebel or resist each fasting period. It is like rewarding the body with normalcy after each fast. There are no set guidelines with respect to how to break the fast. The person can break it any way he chooses. It is for this reason that Eat Stop Eat is especially beneficial for people who eat nutritious food, because no matter how you break the fast, you'll be doing it in a healthy way.

One of the values with the Eat Stop Eat fast is that you're only asking the body to fast for a day at a time, so compliance is relatively easy, compared to other, longer prolonged fasting regimens. Throughout the day of fasting, you know you can look forward to a good meal soon. Pilon does, however, urge moderation, especially for those inclined toward junk or snack foods. The best way to begin an Eat Stop Eat routine, is to try one day of fasting to see how it goes. It does take some discipline, but most people have little trouble adopting it. Eat Stop Eat is a program which, like intraday IF protocols, could be adopted over a long period of time, even throughout one's life. Even if you only fast for one day each week, you'll be able to easily maintain a healthy weight.

The Fast-Feast Approach

The so-called Fast-Feast approach to IF is essentially the same as Eat Stop Eat. The main difference is that it is specifically structured as an ongoing, alternate day routine of feasting one day and fasting the next.

The Fast-Feast fast is more difficult to maintain, since you are continually fasting for 36-hour periods. The program allows for the person to choose any food he wishes to eat on feast days, including junk food and sweets. People who have used the Fast-Feast approach, often report that they quickly lost their cravings for poor food choices on this program.

The Fast-Feast program reaps a fairly rapid weight loss, since the number of calories consumed is nearly cut in half. If you consume 2000 calories on feast days, for example, and you're fasting every other day, then the average number of calories you consume daily is 1000. The biggest risk associated with Fast-Feast is the desire to binge eat on feast days. Feast days need to be strictly limited to a normal day's caloric intake.

The Fast-Feast approach is probably not a practical, long-term dietary strategy. However, once weight loss objectives are realized, they program could be modified to an Eat Stop Eat program, with only one or two days per week of fasting. Since the pattern of fasting every other day has been established with Fast-Feast, switching to only one, or perhaps two days per week of fasting, should be an easy transition.

The Physiology of Eating and Fasting

Understanding the physiological processes behind eating and fasting can be helpful in formulating a personal IF protocol. This knowledge can also be helpful in supporting our motivation and our commitment. It helps to know what's going on inside our bodies as we eat and fast.

The primary physiological objective of an IF program is to cause the body to use its stored energy sources, which include blood sugar and body fat. The process of using these stored reserves is a completely normal process that the human body has evolved to be able to do. Our bodies are built to be able to fast hours, and even days at a time, without any detrimental consequences. Our blood glucose and body fat are reservoirs of energy that we have in place to fuel the body, whenever food is not available. When we fast, we are using these reserves in precisely the way nature intends for them to be used.

When we eat food, we ingest more food energy that we are capable of using right away. Some of this energy from our food is then stored for later use. The hormone insulin is responsible for helping to store this excess energy. The carbohydrates we consume are broken down into individual glucose units, which link together to form glycogen. Glycogen is then stored in the liver and muscle tissue. The body has only a limited amount of space to store glycogen.

When we run out of space to store glycogen, the liver begins to convert glycogen to fat. Some of this fat is retained and stored in the liver, but most of it is distributed to other tissues in the body. This is a relatively complicated process, but there is essentially no limit to how much fat our bodies can store.

When we don't eat for some period of time, insulin levels fall, and this food storage process is reversed. The body first breaks down glycogen into smaller glucose units, and these sugars then are released into the blood. Once that process has run its course, the body must then call on its reserves of fat for its energy.

Tapping our glycogen reserves is the quickest and simplest way to access stored energy. Glycogen gets broken down into glucose, a simpler form of sugar that our body's cells can utilize. Our glycogen reserves can typically provide enough energy to fuel our bodies for 24-36 hours. After the glycogen is used up, the body will begin to tap its fat reserves.

Our bodies are continually moving from the fed, high-insulin state to the fast, low insulin state. We are either in an energy storing mode, or we are in an energy burning mode. It is either one or the other. As long as our eating and fasting periods are balanced, our body weight should not vary that much.

If we begin eating right after we wake up in the morning, and continue to eat continuously throughout the entire day, we remain in the feeding, high-insulin state all day long. This pattern is a certain recipe for weight gain, because we don't give our bodies the opportunity to burn any of its stored fat. Intermittent fasting is a way to ensure that we spend sufficient time in the low-insulin, energy burning state.

Simply put, IF is a solution to the problem of utilizing our body's stored energy reserves, so that they don't accumulate. These reserves are there to be utilized. It's a purely natural process.

Sugar excesses have consequences beyond weight gain and weight retention. Eventually, after we continually add more sugar to our bodies, without subsequently removing those sugars, the excess will build up in the blood and lead to prediabetes or type II diabetes. With the core issue of type II diabetes being the overloading of cells with glucose, then it stands to reason that the way to prevent or mitigate type II diabetes is to engage in a process, IF, that helps remove this excess glucose.

Self-regulating our glucose levels can only be done in one of two ways. We must either consume less sugars and carbohydrates, or engage in activities that utilize and burn these sugars. Fasting is a powerful, yet underutilized method of controlling blood glucose levels. Intermittent fasting is a process that has been scientifically shown to mitigate and reverse type II diabetes without medicines or surgeries. It is not only free, it will actually save you money due to lowering your food bill.

Research into fasting has demonstrated a long list of health and medical benefits, including:

- Loss of weight and body fat
- Reduced blood insulin and glucose levels
- Reduced hemoglobin A1c levels
- Reduced dependency on a variety of medications
- Improved blood pressure

- Improved cholesterol levels
- Improved mental clarity and focus
- Increased energy
- Increased human growth hormone
- Increased longevity
- Cellular cleansing through autophagy activation
- Anti-inflammatory action

Chapter 5

Physiology of Intermittent FASTING

In this chapter, we will explore some of the biological processes and benefits of intermittent fasting. Some of these factors have already been addressed in previous chapters, but in Chapter 5, we will go into greater depth.

Metabolic Syndrome

'Metabolic syndrome' is a term which has been devised to refer to a group of five biological conditions that increase the risk for cardiovascular disease, type II diabetes, and stroke. Metabolic refers to natural physiological processes, including hormonal secretions, that support normal body functions.

The five biological conditions that make up the risk profile of metabolic syndrome are:

1. Belly fat – a large waistline, specifically belly fat, presents a significantly higher risk to heart health than fat accumulation in other parts of the body, such as hips and thighs.
2. High triglyceride levels – triglycerides are fats found in human blood
3. Low HDL cholesterol – HDL cholesterol is referred to as the 'good' cholesterol, because it helps remove cholesterol from arteries.
4. High blood pressure – when blood pressure becomes elevated, and remains elevated over a significant period of time, it causes the heart to work harder than it is designed to work, and can contribute to the build-up of plaque
5. High blood sugar – this includes those diagnosed with type II diabetes, and those with moderately elevated blood sugar, who are diagnosed with prediabetes

It is possible to have any one of these conditions by itself. Having one, or even two of these conditions, does not warrant a metabolic syndrome diagnosis. However, they tend to cluster together. Anyone exhibiting three or more, can be officially diagnosed with metabolic syndrome. Metabolic syndrome quite often includes obesity as one of the three conditions. A lack of adequate physical activity, or sedentary lifestyle, as also a common correlative factor.

With respect to cardiovascular risk, one important factor involves the elasticity of blood vessels, especially arteries that supply the heart with blood. After plaque builds up along the walls of blood vessels, it reduces the diameter of the vessel, and they become rigid, which reduces the heart's blood supply and causes the heart to work harder to pump blood. Plaque is a major cause of high blood pressure, heart damage, heart attacks, and can be potentially life-threatening.

The metabolic syndrome collection of medical conditions makes us more vulnerable to other types of health risks, including infectious diseases, such as viruses. A recently completed study, published online in 2020, confirmed metabolic syndrome risk factors for Covid-19. The researchers commented, in part:

"Many patients with coronavirus disease 2019 (COVID-19) have comorbidities related to metabolic syndrome (MS) during the disease course... MS is a risk factor influencing the progression and prognosis of COVID-2019...Patients with metabolic disorders like obesity, diabetes, cardiovascular and liver disease face a higher risk of infection of COVID-19, greatly affecting the development and prognosis of the disease, being associated with significantly worse outcome in these patients."

Up until June 1, 2020, Brazil had 13,868 reported deaths of Covid-19 infections. Of those deaths, 90% were linked to a comorbidity with metabolic syndrome.

Intermittent Fasting and Hormonal Balance

The endocrine system, as much as any other biological system, controls body fat. Weight loss and healthy weight maintenance are made much easier by optimizing the hormones insulin, ghrelin, and leptin.

Insulin

Insulin is a hormone which is secreted by the pancreas. The pancreas is responsible for:

- Secretion of enzymes into the small intestine which help break down food material, delivered by the stomach
- Production of the hormone insulin, which is secreted into the bloodstream, where it helps to regulate blood glucose

In most American diets, carbohydrates are the main foodstuff which causes insulin levels to rise in our blood. After the body breaks down these complex sugars into glucose, and subsequently releases glucose into our bloodstream, the pancreas releases insulin which serves to deliver these sugars into our cells. A reduction in carbohydrate intake can actually increase insulin sensitivity.

Insulin sensitivity is very important. Resistance to insulin means that our cells are not responding as they should to the hormone. This causes the body to produce higher levels, which causes blood sugar levels to rise, which can then lead to prediabetes and type II diabetes. Insulin resistance also causes a build-up of belly fat, high blood triglycerides, and low HDL (good) cholesterol levels.

Leptin

Leptin is a hormone produced by fat cells. It plays an important role in body weight maintenance by acting upon the hypothalamus to help suppress appetite and to burn fat. Leptin is often thought of as the hunger hormone, or the satisfaction hormone, because it alerts the brain regarding whether or not we've eaten enough. It is considered the master regulator of hunger.

When we eat, leptin is released from our fat cells. When we've eaten enough, it signals the brain that we're full and to stop eating. It tells us if our caloric intake and energy levels are sufficient, or whether we need to continue eating. Several factors are known to influence leptin and ghrelin levels:

- Caloric intake
- Exercise
- Sleep/wake schedule (circadian rhythms)
- Meal timing (circadian rhythms)
- Exposure to natural light
- Stress

When discussing hunger signals and levels, leptin and ghrelin are often mentioned together, since they both respond to essentially the same signals, originating from the stomach and brain. Some important factors about these two hormones are:

- Leptin is generally associated more with eating satisfaction because it helps control appetite.

- Ghrelin is generally associated more with hunger because it tends to increase our desire to eat.
- When our levels of ghrelin and leptin become imbalanced, our pattern of eating when truly hungry, and fasting when satiated, is compromised, leading to fluctuations in our body weight and fat levels.
- Dietary and lifestyle changes that tend to help us regulate leptin, also tend to help control ghrelin levels.

Ghrelin

Ghrelin, the principal appetite stimulator, is released by the stomach. When elevated, it sends signals to the brain that it's time to eat. Several factors can influence our ghrelin secretions, including age, gender, blood glucose levels, and leptin levels. Ghrelin is low and leptin is high before we eat, and ghrelin is high and leptin is low after we eat.

To determine if these two hormones are balanced, we can usually find out from our answers to these questions:

1. Do you tend to eat a lot of processed fast foods and sugary desserts?
2. Do you often find yourself sleep-deprived and/or stressed?
3. Do you consistently undereat?
4. Do you have ongoing food cravings?
5. Are you either overweight or underweight?

If you answered yes to two or more of the above five questions, your leptin/ghrelin hormones are most likely out of balance. If so, intermittent fasting will help restore them to their proper balance and functionality.

Calories and Metabolic Response

One method that scientists use to determine a food's number of calories is to literally burn some of it, and then measure the amount of energy released. Our bodies do not measure calories, and do not respond to any particular number of calories. However, from a metabolic standpoint, 200 calories of broccoli are not equal to 200 calories of sweets.

Our bodies react to the composition of the foods we consume. What is the macronutrient makeup; proteins, fats, and carbohydrates? More importantly, what is the hormonal response to these components? For example, 200 calories of donuts will cause a spike in blood sugar, which will elicit a corresponding insulin response. However, 200 calories of spinach will not cause such a response.

A common misperception with respect to our metabolism of food is that all calories are equal; calories in and calories out. They are not equal. Controlling our body weight by merely controlling caloric intake is not a winning strategy. Hormonal response to the foods we consume is a more critical factor than caloric intake alone.

Since the 1970's, we have evolved from a three-meal-a-day culture to a six-meal-a-day culture. This perpetual onslaught of carbs and sugars creates insulin resistance. Fat cells enlarge and trigger the constant release of leptin. When we stimulate this release of leptin too often, it leads to leptin resistance.

Body Weight Homeostasis

Homeostasis is the tendency toward a state of equilibrium between interdependent elements and processes. In biology, it refers to an equilibrium between physiological processes and systems. It is the steady internal state of ideal physical and chemical conditions, including variables such as body temperature, fluid balances, and hormonal levels.

As an analogy, you can think of homeostasis as a thermostat. When set to 72 degrees, it will seek this temperature. If the temperature rises above 72, it will trigger the air conditioner. If the temperature falls below 72, it will trigger the heater.

We have an inner mechanism that helps regulate our body weight. Our bodies have a predetermined weight that is innately preferred. We may not think of this weight as our ideal weight. If we've been 20 pounds overweight for a long period of time, the body thinks that this is our preferred weight. Our bodies attempt to defend this body weight, or homeostasis, by burning off more calories when we accumulate too much fat, in an attempt to return to this preferred weight. When we lose too much weight, our bodies burn less calories to compensate.

When we gain too much body fat, our fat cells enlarge and release leptin. When leptin reaches the brain, it tells us that we have accumulated too much fat, and our appetite is turned down. Then, after eating less, our insulin level subsides.

What happens in weight gain is that there is no lack of leptin. There is, however, a lack of response on our part. We ignore the signals our body is providing and continue to eat. We break this back-and-forth (thermostatic) loop and accumulate fat. The best way to reset this back-and-forth process is to reduce insulin levels for a sufficient amount of time to lower these leptin levels. Insulin, therefore, is the key to balancing these hormonal levels, and to setting our bodies back on a course toward healthy weight management. This can be a short-term fix, or a long-term process, depending on our weight and hormonal health.

Fasting, especially intermittent fasting, is an effective way to achieve caloric reduction. It is also an effective means of optimizing insulin, ghrelin, and leptin to help the body build lean body mass. When insulin levels drop enough, the body switches fuel sources from food to glycogen, and once glycogen is depleted, fat. Since there is plenty of fat reserves available, the process is seamless, with our metabolic rates maintained. The fat-burning process is known as lipolysis. It is a metabolic process that transforms triglycerides by hydrolyzing them into glycerol and fatty acids. It also helps utilize stored energy during fasting and exercise.

During fasting, as insulin levels fall, the body reacts with a hormonal surge. These hormones include adrenaline, human growth hormone, and cortisol. They assist the liver in releasing its stored glucose, and they increase our metabolic rate.

On longer, alternate day fasting protocols, after the first 16 hours, glycogen stores in our liver are tapped. These stores will last 24 to 36 hours. During this period, the body will also target and eliminate unneeded or damaged proteins. Growth hormone increases fairly dramatically, as much as 300% on a shorter, one day fast, and as much as 500% on a prolonged fast of three days or longer.

During refeeding, the lost proteins will be rebuilt with new, healthy proteins. This same process can also target damaged cells, including brain and nerve cells, through a cellular process known as autophagy. Intermittent fasting is a superior method of developing and maintaining lean body mass compared to dieting and calorie cutting. Crash diets retard metabolic rates, rather than managing insulin to enhance fat burning.

Carbs and Other Food Choices

There are a number of ethnic diets around the world that are high in carbohydrates, yet the people consuming those diets do not develop obesity. It is possible to eat high-carbohydrate content foods and still maintain healthy insulin levels.

The difference is that these ethnic groups maintain a 3-meal-a-day dietary routine, rather than eating 6 meals or more, and they eat little or no sugar. Sugar is far more fattening than carbohydrates. Fructose, for example, is about twenty times as fattening as eating bread. Refined and processed grains also have little effect on satisfying hunger, because it is the fat, protein, and fiber, which are removed, that induce satiety.

Type II Diabetes

Type II diabetes is treated, by many physicians, by increasing insulin levels. But this is a flawed treatment strategy, because it just serves to increase glucose levels in the liver. This sugar either turns into fat, or it circulates through the blood to our tissues and organs. Over time, the body rots with all the sugar everywhere, perpetually, which is a major reason why diabetics are more susceptible to infectious diseases.

Elevated blood glucose is not the cause of type II diabetes, but rather a symptom. By targeting blood glucose, the physician is treating the symptom, not the disease. A person with type II diabetes has too much sugar already. He should eat a low carbohydrate diet, with little to no refined sugars. Excess sugars should be burnt off with intermittent fasting. Type II diabetes, for most patients, can be reversed through intermittent fasting.

Type II diabetes is just one example of conflicts of interest that can develop within the medical system. Supposedly, medical science is an evidence-based system. But if our evidence becomes corrupted, then our medical protocols become corrupted too. Much of our scientific, research-based evidence is produced by pharmaceutical companies. Since much of the funding for medical research within universities comes from the private sector; i.e. large corporations, shoddy research is too often the outcome. Scientists are not immune to bias. Special interests need to be removed from the research process for the benefit of all.

Caloric Restriction and Longevity

The PubMed database contains over 9500 research studies that address 'caloric restriction'. Many of these studies are focused specifically on caloric restriction itself, showing evidence of its effectiveness in treating many health conditions. These conditions include:

- Depression
- Cancer prevention and treatment
- Longevity
- Metabolic disorders
- Obesity
- Cognitive benefits
- Bladder dysfunction
- Chronic kidney disease
- Muscle strength and physical performance
- Type II diabetes
- Heart failure

Caloric restriction is one of the only therapeutic models that is widely recognized to be effective in increasing lifespan and healthspan. However, the research concluded to date is primarily animal research, using both mice and monkeys as test subjects. Due to human lifespan being now close to eighty years, it will take a bit of time to assess human longevity research on caloric restriction.

There is, however, a serum test which has been devised to evaluate a person's 'internal age'; the actual relative age of your physiology, as opposed to your calendar age. The test, known as the 'Inside Tracker', was developed by a team of Harvard scientists, including the well-known longevity researcher, Dr. David Sinclair.

Inside Tracker has been specifically devised to evaluate certain biological markers, known to influence longevity. The test is especially valuable to researchers conducting work on human longevity, because they can use it to evaluate a certain protocol's effectiveness in extending human life. They don't have to wait for an entire human lifespan to be completed. They can devise a test over a shorter period; six months, for example. They can then measure these longevity-related biomarkers at the end of the testing period, and compare data to their controls.

CR has traditionally been achieved by slashing food intake. This has been a problem in conducting human trials, due to lack of compliance by test subjects. Reducing calories over a shorter, fixed period of time is not difficult to do. But if you ask a person to reduce the size of all of his meals for the remainder of his life, total compliance is unrealistic. Just imagine every meal portion being reduced by one third, forever. With mice and monkeys, it's easy to do. You just give them less food. What are they going to do about it? They're in cages.

The bright side is that, for those animals who do participate in CR research, their health is often improved and their lifespans are extended. Of course, if you're living in a cage every day of your life, maybe you don't want your life extended.

Dr. Sinclair's Harvard team has dug deep into the process of human aging, investigating longevity on genetic and cellular levels. Aging is now known to be associated with compromised DNA. They've identified a common protein, known as DBC1, that interferes with DNA repair. The underlying problem appears to be caused by a reduction of a cellular chemical known as NAD. NAD levels decrease with age. When we're younger, and our NAD levels are high, DBC1 does not interfere with DNA repair. Dr. Sinclair believes that aging begins with compromised DNA, resulting in large part from decreased levels of NAD.

NAD protects DNA through its ability to stimulate a group of seven proteins known as 'sirtuins'. Sirtuins are involved in a variety of biological processes, including aging. More importantly, sirtuins are produced and activated during periods of caloric restriction. This includes all types of fasting, especially intermittent fasting.

Sirtuins are known to protect chromosomes and stem cells. They also protect cells from the harmful inflammatory effects of decayed senescent cells. Scientists are busy trying to devise drugs and supplements that will help mimic the cellular activity of caloric restriction.

For now, the best way to activate sirtuins, from the standpoint of both effectiveness and compliance, is with intermittent fasting. When a person fasts, the body increases production of an enzyme known as NAMPT. NAMPT is essential in the synthesis of NAD. Researchers have concluded that increasing NAMPT levels through fasting is an effective way to increase human lifespan.

Caloric Restriction Research

Caloric restriction, abbreviated CR, is sometimes referred in research papers as 'dietary restriction', and abbreviated DR. Studies conducted on rodents have shown as much as a 40% increase in lifespan through the application of a life-long reduction in calories. This level of increase appears to correlate directly with the amount of caloric restriction imposed on the animals.

This longevity response to caloric restriction has been discovered in every animal species tested to date. However, researchers believe that some species react to it more favorably than others. This response probably evolved ages ago, as a way to increase the chances for survival during times of seasonal famines or other periodic food shortages. For a smaller animal, like a mouse, who lives only a few years, a seasonal famine represents a much greater portion of his lifespan. For this reason, his response to a food shortage has apparently evolved in a much more dramatic way.

CR testing on primates is important in order to have some means to gauge its potential effects on human aging. A 2014 study, published in "Nature Communications", demonstrated the effects of CR on adult monkeys. Each of the test monkeys had his food intake decreased 10% for three consecutive months, to arrive at their target of 30% caloric reduction. The control monkeys were fed a normal diet throughout their entire adult lives.

Researchers divided all of the animals into groups, based on the cause of death. In the control group, who were fed a normal diet, 63% of the monkeys died of age-related causes. This compares with only 26% of the monkeys in the CR group dying of age-related causes. Researchers also discovered that of the monkeys who died of non-age-related-causes, the CR monkeys live significantly longer lives. At 27 years, all of the control monkeys had died, compared to over 50% of the test monkeys who were still alive. 20% lived more than 30 years, which is considered a long lifespan for a monkey. Researchers were also able to measure benefits in the general health and function of the CR animals, compared to the control group.

One human study, a.k.a. the CALERIE study, which was conducted over a twelve year period, reported in their conclusion:

> *"CR completely protects against high blood pressure, atherosclerosis/ coronary heart disease and diabetes, and that the middle-aged and older CR society members in our study appear 20 to 30 yrs younger than their chronological ages in terms of their cardiovascular elasticity, and heart rate variability and gene expression profile in muscle (i.e. markers of aging)."*

They went on to add:

"It has also become very evident from our experience with the CAL-ERIE study that the great majority of people find CR to be extremely difficult and not feasible long-term."

So, we know from these and other studies that CR will support overall health and make you biologically younger, but we still don't know with certainty just how much it will extend human lifespan. More importantly, it is going to be extremely challenging for any human research into CR to maintain compliance amongst test subjects. How many people are willing to cut down their caloric intake by 30% for the remainder of their lives?

Intermittent Fasting to the Rescue

The same researchers who conducted the CALERIE study cited above, recommend that some form of intermittent fasting should be utilized in order to achieve test subject compliance, since long-term CR is not a practical way to achieve a significant reduction in caloric intake. They believed that IF would be much easier to adhere to, while garnering similar results.

When they substituted IF for a 30% CR protocol in obese test subjects, they had very positive results with biomarkers related to aging. Their IF regimen was a water fast for two days each week.

Another IF approach, formulated by an English doctor named Walter Longo, resulted in high compliance with test subjects. His work has been published in the journal, "Cell Metabolism". He had them consume a low-calorie diet for five consecutive days each month. His diet reduced caloric intake by 34% to 54% of normal, with a specific list of acceptable foods, including proteins, carbohydrates, fats, and micronutrients. These same test subjects ate normally on the rest of the days of the month. After just three months, test subjects had lowered risk factors and biomarkers for aging, diabetes, cancer, and cardiovascular disease.

Dr. Longo's protocol was not an IF protocol, in the strictest sense, since people did eat during the 'fasting periods', but his system still managed to achieve some highly significant results.

Chapter 6

The Intermittent Fasting for Life Method

"Adopt the IFL Method for life. Make it a part of who you are."

This chapter is devoted to presenting the "Intermittent Fasting for Life Method". This IF method has been devised and formulated after reviewing and consolidating all of the best intermittent fasting methods already discussed previously in this book. Also taken into account in devising the IFL Method are dozens of research studies that address fasting and caloric deprivation.

The Psychology of Fasting

By now, you've read enough to be convinced that fasting is a healthy practice to incorporate into your life, and that intermittent fasting is the easiest and most practical way for most people to fast. Fasting is essential. We need to fast. We have evolved through natural processes to have fasting be a necessary component to a long, healthy life.

Now, the hard part; doing it.

Actually, adopting intermittent fasting doesn't have to be difficult. There is only one thing standing in your way; your mind.

You have trained your mind to eat when you experience hunger pangs. You have also trained your mind to eat continually, whether you're hungry or not. How many times have you eaten a meal or a snack when you weren't actually hungry? Too often, we eat out of boredom or out of habit. Sometimes we eat solely because it is socially expedient to eat. Unfortunately, this pattern of continual eating and snacking, even when we're not hungry, has become a feature of the American way of life. As a result, obesity has now become a feature of the American landscape.

Retraining the Mind

Your mind doesn't want you to be thin. Your mind doesn't want you to be fat. Your mind doesn't really care what you do, as long as it has a pattern of repetitive thinking and behavior to follow. The mind is like a horse. Horses need a leader. Your mind needs a leader, and that leader is you.

The reason that your mind reacts to hunger urges by eating food is because you've programmed it to react that way. The reason that you snack between meals is that you've established snacking as a pattern of behavior. The reason why you eat late is because the mind has grown accustomed to the habit of eating late.

If you want to reap the benefits of intermittent fasting, the mind must be reprogrammed with new patterns of thinking and behavior. The mind can be a powerful ally in any human endeavor. It can also stand in your way when you make attempts to transform your life in a new, positive way.

Research has shown that it takes from two weeks to two months for a new habit to be formed. If you are to establish new patterns of feeding and fasting, then it will take some effort in the beginning. But after a few weeks, after sufficient repetition, the mind will get on board with the new program and support your efforts toward self-improvement.

Your Three IF Commitments

There are three commitments that are absolutely necessary for any person to make if he wants to incorporate intermittent fasting into his or her lifestyle going forward. These things are:

1. FORM NEW HABITS

The only way IF will ever work for you is if you recognize the fact that, for the first few weeks or so, the mind will rebel. It doesn't like change. Establishing your new patterns of feeding and fasting will take some effort and some time. But after two weeks, your new routine will become easier, and eventually will become habitual. From that point forward, the mind will fully support your IF protocol.

2. EMBRACE HUNGER

As soon as you embark on your IF journey, you will begin to experience hunger. This experience must be embraced. You need to allow yourself to become hungry without reacting to this feeling by eating. Instead, react to it by intentionally not eating. Drink a glass of water.

There are two components to hunger; a physiological one, and a mental one. The physical component is created by the hormones insulin, ghrelin, and leptin. The levels of these hormones do, at times, cause an aching in the belly. This aching cannot be avoided. The second component to hunger is mental. The mental feature has to do with how you think about hunger, and how you react to these gnawing feelings.

Get used to this feeling. It's a good experience, not a bad experience. Every time you feel hungry, say to yourself; "My IF program is working now. I'm burning glucose and fat. I'm cleaning my body out. I'm losing weight."

When you adopt an IF program of any kind, experiencing hunger is unavoidable. When you feel it during the day, be thankful that your body is mending and thinning down. After you learn to simply ignore it and let it be there, your mind will stop reacting to it by wanting to eat. Allow hunger to be your 'new normal'.

3. STOP SNACKING

You simply cannot retain the habit of between-meal snacking if you're going to adopt an IF protocol successfully. Snacking has to go. Eliminating snacking is Intermittent Fasting rule #1. A snack is a meal. Limit your daily meals to three. If you snack, it's one of your three daily meals. Even if the snack is small, it interrupts your metabolic processes. You switch gears from burning sugar and fat to accumulating sugar and fat. (the IFL Method does allow for some limited snacking and cheating)

So, these three things; being patient and steadfast while new habits are formed, embracing hunger, and eliminating snacking are absolute prerequisites for adopting IF into your lifestyle. If you are not prepared to make these three commitments, it would be best to forgo IF for the time being until a more advantageous time presents itself when you can make these commitments.

The Intermittent Fasting for Life Method

The Intermittent Fasting for Life Method is flexible, and allows each person the ability tailor it to their own lifestyle, diet, and personal health objectives. It includes the following components:

- Acceptance of the feeling of hunger as being normal
- Commitment to eliminate snacking
- Commitment to adherence to the IFL Method 90% of the time
- An introductory experimental period
- Adopt 15:9 for life
- Delayed light breakfast – 9:00 AM – 10:30 AM (early juice OK)
- Midday meal largest of the day, if feasible
- Dinner by 6:00 PM and no later than 7:30 PM
- Weekends try to maintain IF eating schedule

- Weekend carb/sweet cheat allowed
- Prolonged 36-hour water-only fast once weekly until weight objective is surpassed by 4-5 pounds. (juice, herb tea, and broth alternatives)
- General nutritional guidelines
- Dietary supplementation
- General workout and activity guidelines

The Introductory Period

Once you've made the commitments to eliminate snacking and embrace the feeling of hunger, an introductory period of five to seven days is recommended to begin your IFL Method program. The purpose of this period is to experience hunger, and especially to experience allowing those feelings to be there.

During this period, the only changes you will make to your fast/feed routine are;

- You will eat an early dinner, no later than 6:30 PM
- You will not eat any other solid food until you retire for bed

After your evening meal has been completed, you may drink water or herb tea only. Before continuing with the rest of the IFL program, follow these two simple introductory guidelines for a minimum of five days continuously. Once you've accomplished this initial task, you're ready to begin.

Establish Objectives

If you have a particular goal, or set of goals in mind that you want to achieve with your intermittent fasting, write them down. Are you targeting a particular body weight? Write it down. Is there some other health objective you're trying to achieve? Perhaps you want to improve your metabolic numbers, like cholesterol, blood pressure, or blood glucose. If so, write it all down.

If you are targeting a specific weight, it is best to go beyond your weight objective by four or five pounds. The reason for going lower than your weight goal is that, human nature being what it is, you may want to slack off a little on your routine as a way to celebrate your achievement. This typically involves a modest weight gain of a few pounds. Plan for this by exceeding your weight objective before you celebrate.

15:9 For Life

The IFL Method is an adaptation of the 16:8 protocol, but with the feeding window expanded each day by one hour. The main reason to expand the feed window is to accommodate the daily schedules that contemporary Americans tend to follow. A nine-hour window is simply more practical for most people to adapt to, in part because many people work eight-hour jobs. The one-hour reduction of the fasting window will have a negligible effect on results.

So, if the first meal of the day is at 7:00 AM, the final meal of the day is consumed no later than 4:00 PM. On the other hand, if the first meal of the day is consumed at 10:00 AM, then the final meal of the day is consumed no later than 7:00 PM. Remember, no snacking between meals. Whatever it is you want to eat at that time of the day, eat it all together at one time. Between meals, drink water, tea, or coffee. Don't load your tea and coffee up with rich creamers and sugar. If you want to use a sweetener, use stevia. Stevia is plant-based and contains no calories.

The intention of the 15:9 IF protocol is for it to be adopted for life. Once the habit is established, there is no reason not to. This is the optimal fast/feed schedule that our bodies want and need. By adopting 15:9 over a period of time, one to two months for example, you will experience a slow, but steady weight loss. At some point, your body weight will reach a state of equilibrium, or homeostasis. This weight is most likely your target weight. When you reach this weight, your body will tend to defend this weight, as being its preferred weight.

However, if you still haven't quite reached your target weight, getting the rest of the way there is fairly simple to do. You've already established your 15:9 habit. Now, it's just a matter of making some adjustments with your caloric intake. When you're firmly on the 15:9 schedule, it won't take much caloric adjustment to get the remaining unwanted weight off.

Breakfast

There is one point of view in the field of nutrition that breakfast is the most important meal of the day and should also be the largest. But this approach to eating doesn't conform to our hormonal circadian rhythms. The hormone ghrelin, which is the hormone that causes appetite, is at its lowest levels of the day at 8:00 AM. Why not take advantage of this with a light, late breakfast?

On the 15:9 fast/feed schedule, you will need to buy time somewhere. This time can only be found early in the day or late in the day. Since ghrelin is low in the morning, causing your appetite to be under control, the best period of the day to buy this time is in the morning. If you can delay breakfast until 9:00 AM, then dinner can be pushed to 6:00 PM. If you delay breakfast to 10:00 AM, then dinner can be pushed to 7:00 PM.

From a practical standpoint, you may need something in your system earlier than 9:00 AM to get 'jump-started'. It that's the case, have a glass of fresh juice. One glass of juice at 7:00 AM or 7:30 AM will not interfere with your 15:9 daily fast/feed metabolic schedule.

If you work full-time, hopefully you're in a situation where you can munch on a light breakfast as you begin your workday. This is an area in the IFL program where you may need to be somewhat creative. Ask yourself: "Given my work environment and routine, how can I devise a light, nutritious breakfast that I can eat at my work station around

9:00 AM?" Most workers have some coffee to start their workday, and many workers combine that coffee with some kind of snack.

The Midday Meal or Lunch

The midday meal can be consumed at any time that is convenient to your schedule. If possible, this should be your largest meal of the day. However, it may not be practical to make this your primary daily meal. If the midday meal is not your largest meal, then it should be comparable to your evening meal. Remember, once this meal is consumed, no snacking.

Dinner

Your final meal of the day should ideally be consumed by 6:00 PM, but never later than 7:30 PM. Once this meal is completed, your fasting period begins. For the rest of the evening, until you retire for bed, drink only pure water or tea.

Weekends

The IFL Method calls for a two-day period each week that allows for some relaxation in the fast/feed schedule and dietary choices. This two-day period may be the weekend, Saturday and Sunday, or it may be some other two-day period that better fits your personal routine. During these two days, your pattern of work and leisure may be different. These may be your days off from work. You may have some televised events you want to watch, like sports. You may want to grab a bag of chips and some salsa and munch while you watch.

As long as you don't binge, having a little break from your fast/feed routine won't create a set-back. During your weekend, you may also want to relax your carbohydrate intake with some pasta or mashed potatoes. Again, don't binge. It's comfort food. Be comfortable. Then, on Monday morning, hop back onto your 15:9 schedule.

It isn't necessary to take this little break each week. It's optional. If you would prefer not to relax your IFL routine during your weekend, then don't.

One-Day Prolonged Water Fasts

After you've been on the 15:9 fast/feed schedule for a few weeks or a month, there is another powerful component that you can add. This component is a one-day, water-only fast. It is an optional component to the IFL Method, but a powerful one, and one that will accelerate your weight loss objectives.

The one-day fast is actually a 36-hour fast. It begins on the evening of day #1, after you've consumed your final meal of that day. The fast continues throughout the next day, with only water or tea being consumed. Then, on breakfast of day #3, you break your one-day fast with a healthy, nutritious meal.

The one-day fast is actually a short, prolonged fast. During the fasting day, the hormone ghrelin will still be secreted, so you will feel hungry. After a prolonged fast of two days, ghrelin levels drop off sharply, but on a one-day fast, you will experience hunger. By this time, you already have some experience with hunger, so this shouldn't be a problem.

There is no set schedule for utilizing the one-day fast. You could do it once. You could do it once per week. The more often you incorporate the one-day fast into your 15:9 routine, the faster you'll reach your health objective(s). The one-day fast is your accelerator. If you do it once per month, you push the accelerator down one-quarter of the way. If you do it twice per month, you push the accelerator down half-way. If you do it every week, you have the accelerator pushed down to the floor.

When you schedule your one-day fast, do it on a day when you don't anticipate a heavy load of physical activity. Your day could be a weekend day, or a day during the week. But relative to your personal schedule, it is your most opportune day to do it.

The one-day fast can also be modified by including a low caloric intake of juices, smoothies, or soups. This may be desirable if it is your first attempt at the one-day fast, or if you feel like you need some caloric intake on that particular day.

Nutritional Choices

The IFL Method does not require you to make any broad changes with respect to the foods you normally eat. Except for possibly eliminating a few obviously harmful choices, just maintain the same diet you normally eat now. After you've put all of your effort into embracing hunger and forgoing snacking, you don't want to sabotage your achievement by loading up on unhealthy, non-nutritious foods. Be nice to yourself.

Your main source of junky food is most likely going to be in the category of carbohydrates. We need some carbohydrates, but there are good, beneficial carbohydrates and there are unhealthy carbs.

The good carbs are obtained from whole, unprocessed grains. Brown rice, bananas, and whole oats, for example, are excellent choices. A sugary donut, for example, is a poor choice. Pastas, chips, and white bread are also poor choices. If you want to 'cheat' a little on your weekend days with these carbs, that's okay, as long as they're consumed in moderation. Whatever you do, don't backslide by reestablishing a new (old) habit of overeating carbohydrates.

You have four distinct food groups to choose from:

1. Fresh fruits and vegetables = 50%
2. Proteins = 25%
3. Fats = 15%
4. Carbohydrates = 10%

Try to follow these general percentages as closely as possible. However, you don't need to carry around a calculator and a calorie-counting table. This doesn't need to be scientifically tracked. This is just a general guideline to keep in mind when preparing your meal plans.

Nutritional Supplementation

The field of dietary supplementation has come a long way since vitamin and mineral supplements were first introduced in the 1940's. It has become a sophisticated, highly scientific field. There is now a huge body of scientific literature available that pertains to the effectiveness of hundreds of dietary supplements.

There are some dietary supplements which are so important, that practically everyone either needs them, or can benefit from them. A short list of these supplements includes:

Green Superfood Powders –

Green superfoods, like spirulina, wheat grass powder, and barley grass powder contain an incredibly high concentration of nutrients. Wheat grass powder, for example, contains practically every important nutritional ingredient there is. Everyone can benefit from consuming these types of supplements. Add them to juice or a smoothie, because their high chlorophyl content produces some mild bitterness.

Omege-3 Fatty Acids

The scientifically established benefits from consuming omega-3's are numerous. They are especially important for maintaining a healthy heart and metabolism. Omega-3's are usually derived from fish oils. However, they are also obtained from algal oil. The reason that omega-3's are found in high concentrations in fish is that fish eat algae. So, algae (algal oil) is the source of omega-3's for the fish.

Vitamin D

Nearly half of Americans are deficient in Vitamin D. We work and play indoors, and don't get enough time out in the sun each day. Vitamin D deficiency has been scientifically linked to weight gain and obesity. Make sure you're getting enough vitamin D. Get outdoors in the sun each day for at least twenty minutes, or supplement your diet.

Protein Supplement

Most people don't need a protein supplement. The amount of protein they consume in their normal diets is sufficient. However, there are some people who can benefit from protein supplementation. If you do strenuous physical work, you're engaged in some form of athletic training, or you have adopted a strenuous fitness routine, you probably need some extra protein. You may also want to supplement if you believe that your normal diet may not contain enough protein.

Protein supplement powders can be mixed with water, juice, or added to smoothies. Pea and whey are good sources of natural protein. Soy is a good choice for women, because along with the protein, there will most likely also be some increased estrogen, since soy contains phytoestrogens.

Workouts and Activity Levels

Regardless of why you are considering intermittent fasting, you must always include physical training and activity into your lifestyle. Physical activity burns calories, and has a myriad of other health-related benefits associated with it. If you're attempting to lose weight, you absolutely must be physically active. Your activity level should be appropriate to your age and overall physical condition. But activity of some kind is an absolute requirement for weight loss and for maintaining a healthy heart and healthy metabolism.

90% Commitment Objective

Some people who adopt the IFL Method will find it fairly easy to follow, once they've established the necessary routine and fast/feed habits. However, most people will have periods of time, such as their weekend days, when they will relax their adherence. That's alright, as long as you're not completely thrown off track. If you make a commitment to following the method's guidelines at least 90% of the time, you will still have 100% success. If might prolong the time it takes you to realize your healing/weight loss goals, but you'll still get there.

Adopt the IFL Method for life. Make it a part of who you are.

The Intermittent Fasting for Life Checklist:

Below is a chart that you can use to refer to, and to remind yourself of your objectives and your commitment. When you begin the program, after you've read each of the listed items, place your initials next to the appropriate factor. Keep this checklist handy and, as a reminder, refer to it often.

YOUR INITIALS	MY INTERMITTENT FASTING OBJECTIVES AND COMMITMENTS
	My objectives for adopting intermittent fasting are as follows: BODY WEIGHT OBJECTIVE: OTHER HEALTH OBJECTIVES:
	I understand that successful intermittent fasting will require my accepting the feeling of hunger as being normal.
	I understand that successful intermittent fasting will require that I stop all snacking between meals.
	I will begin my intermittent fasting with a trial period where my objective is to water-fast for five consecutive days from the end of each evening meal to bedtime.
	I will adopt a 15:9 fast/feed schedule, in which I will adhere to a nine-hour feed window every day.

YOUR INITIALS	MY INTERMITTENT FASTING OBJECTIVES AND COMMITMENTS
	I will attempt to take advantage of my circadian hormonal patterns by eating a light, late breakfast each day.
	I will make healthy food choice decisions, with an emphasis on fresh fruits and vegetables, and whole grain carbohydrates.
	I will maintain a healthy and practical routine of physical activity.
	If and when appropriate and desirable, I will conduct periodic one-day water-only fasts to enhance and accelerate my fasting objectives.
	I understand that if I maintain my intermittent fasting protocols at a 90% level, that I will have 100% success.

Chapter 7

Intermittent Fasting Research

Scientific Research in Nutrition and Fasting

The National Library of Medicine, a division of The National Institutes of Health, has an online database, PubMed, with over thirty million published research studies conducted all over the world in just about every field of health science imaginable.

https://pubmed.ncbi.nlm.nih.gov/

Most of this research was conducted over the past 40 years or so, but some studies date to the early twentieth century. The majority of these studies were originally published in one of the many biomedical journals around the world, both in print and online. Some originate from books and other similar databases.

Anyone who wants to do their own research into any health-related issue can easily do so. The PubMed site has a good search engine, so if you're looking for studies on intermittent fasting, for example, you just need to type it in and click 'search'. After searching for 'intermittent fasting', your search results will yield over 123,000 studies that contain the words, 'intermittent fasting', somewhere in the study. If you search just the term 'fasting', your search will yield over 132,000 results. Needless to say, there has been an enormous amount of research conducted, which in some way or other, involves fasting or intermittent fasting.

When you look through search results, read each result carefully to determine whether you believe that the study may have the information you're looking for. You can always narrow your search. For example, if you are curious whether or not intermittent fasting can have anti-inflammatory effects, then search for 'intermittent fasting inflammation'. The PubMed search engine will return about 5500 results.

Reading Research Studies

The research studies found in PubMed are written by scientists. Scientists, like medical doctors, have their own language of anatomical, physiological, and scientific terms, which lay people are largely unfamiliar with. Therefore, when reading PubMed research, it is important to do so with a dictionary nearby, because you will need to refer to it as you read. Your dictionary could be, of course, your google search engine, which will yield you definitions at the speed of light. Often the words you want to have clarified, wind up relating to some relatively simple health concept that most people are familiar with. You will probably think to yourself, "It would be a lot easier to read this if they would just use common terminology". You will not be the first person to have had this reaction. Regardless, keep your dictionary close at hand.

Some of the research studies are complete studies. They contain the entire study, with charts and lots of specifics on testing parameters and outcomes. There are other studies that only contain the 'abstract'. The abstract is just that; an edited down version that usually only contains a description of the study and the conclusions drawn by the authors of the study. Often the information you want or need is available in the abstract. If not, you will need to find the information you want within the full study. You can save time by following this protocol:

1. Read the title
2. Read the first three to five sentences to determine the objectives and scope of the study.
3. Determine if the study involved was just a lab study, was it an animal study, or was it a human trial?
4. Go to near the end of the study and read the results section.
5. Then, read the conclusion section, which usually follow the results.

After reading these sections, you will have determined whether or not the study was relative to your needs, and most likely, you'll have the answers you sought in the first place.

Another important issue to remember with respect to scientific research is that not all of these studies agree. In fact, disagreement between scientists is commonplace. Why?

One reason that research outcomes differ is due to intent. The researcher was seeking a particular outcome. It is not difficult to cause a predetermined outcome in a health-related study. It is normally done by structuring the parameters of the study in a way that will ensure a certain outcome. For example, if you're trying to demonstrate the ineffectiveness of a particular herbal extract, you can use a very weak concentration of the extract in your study. In the written text of the study itself, all that is needed for the researcher to state is that they used a 'standardized extract'. Of course, standardized herbal extracts can have a concentration of 5% of the active ingredient, or they can have a 95% concentration of this ingredient. A 95% concentration is twenty times more potent than a 5% concentration.

Therefore, it is always wise to investigate who sponsored the study. If it was sponsored by a manufacturer, or a trade association, then the study may not be as valid as a study conducted by a university or research institution using public funding.

With respect to studies conducted on fasting or intermittent fasting, the results and conclusions of pertinent studies should be highly valid, compared to studies on drugs, foods and supplement ingredients. Since there is no manufacturer or trade association that benefits from the results of a study on not-eating, there is no commercial entity that stands to gain or lose from these studies' outcomes.

Study #1

Effects of intermittent fasting on body composition and clinical health markers in humans

Research review studies are analyses that are conducted by scientists who collect all available research on a particular subject and then pool all of the data together, in an attempt to obtain a broader and more accurate picture of a particular research query. This study was one such study, published in 2015 by the International Life Sciences Institute.

While the study looked at data from several IF protocols, the alternate-day fasting data provided the most reliable and accurate information. With respect to a variety of health markers, in trials lasting from three to twelve weeks, the researchers found:

1. A reduction in body weight of between 3% to 7%
2. A reduction in body fat from 6.6 pounds to 12 pounds
3. A reduction in cholesterol from 10% to 21%
4. A reduction in triglycerides from 14% to 42%

In trials lasting from twelve to twenty-four weeks, researchers found:

1. A reduction in body weight of between 3% to 9%
2. A reduction in body fat from 3% to 9%
3. A 5% to 20% reduction in cholesterol
4. A 17% to 50% reduction in triglycerides

Study #2

Alternate-day fasting, in nonobese subjects: effects on body weight, body composition, and energy metabolism

The purpose of this study was to determine whether or not alternate-day fasting was an effective way to improve biomarkers associated with aging and longevity. Sixteen healthy, nonobese subjects were selected; eight men, and eight women. The group fasted every other day for twenty-two days. Researchers measured the following:

1. Body weight
2. Body composition
3. Resting metabolic rate
4. Respiratory quotient
5. Body temperature
6. Blood glucose
7. Insulin
8. Free fatty acids
9. Ghrelin hormone levels and appetite

The study showed the following results:

1. Subjects lost 2.5% of their initial body weight
2. Subjects lost 4% of their initial fat mass
3. Hunger levels increased on the first day and remained elevated throughout the testing period
4. Resting metabolic rate and respiratory quotient did not change
5. Fat burning increased
6. Insulin levels decreased significantly; 57% lower

The study concluded that ADF was an effective weight maintenance and weight loss protocol for nonobese subjects, with a significant increase in fat burning. The principal drawback they saw was that hunger levels did not subside on fasting days, likely making the program a difficult one for many people to comply with.

Study #3

Early Time-Restricted Feeding Improves Insulin Sensitivity, Blood Pressure, and Oxidative Stress Even without Weight Loss in Men with Prediabetes

The authors of this study conceded at the outset that there have been numerous studies which have demonstrated the health-related benefits of intermittent fasting. These benefits include improved insulin sensitivity, improved blood pressure, and lower oxidative stress. However, one question which has been raised is whether or not these favorable outcomes resulted from the IF protocol, or were they actually the secondary effects of the weight loss experienced by the test subjects.

The IF protocol used in this case is called 'early time-restricted feeding, or eTRF. Early time-restricted feeding is a fast/feed schedule which begins every morning at around 8:00 AM and ends at 2:00 PM. In other words, it's a six-hour feeding window, with the largest and final meal of the day being consumed in the early to mid-afternoon.

In this particular study, a group of adult men with prediabetes was divided randomly into two groups. One group went on a strict 6-hour eTRF protocol. The control group maintained a 12-hour eating window, followed by a 12-hour fast, with eating commencing at 8:00 AM and ending at 8:00 PM each day. Both groups were fed identical diets, specifically designed to allow all participants to steadily maintain their weight throughout the 5-week test period. The study was scrupulously monitored to ensure compliance.

Researchers measured four areas:

1. Glucose tolerance, post-meal insulin spikes, and insulin sensitivity
2. Cardiovascular risk factors
3. Markers for oxidative stress and inflammation
4. Metabolic hormones

During the five-week test period, both groups maintained their standard body weights, so researchers knew that their results were not caused by weight loss.

Their results demonstrated the following:

1. eTRF reduced insulin levels and improved insulin sensitivity and immune response
2. eTRF lowered blood pressure
3. eTRF had no measurable effect on cholesterol levels or arterial stiffness
4. eTRF reduced oxidative stress, but had no effect on inflammatory markers
5. eTRF reduced evening ghrelin secretion levels, resulting in reduced evening appetite

The study's researchers concluded that IF, especially an IF protocol that was focused on early eating patterns, in line with our metabolic circadian rhythms, is an especially effective intervention for prediabetes and prehypertension patients.

Study #4

When less may be more: calorie restriction and response to cancer therapy

In this study, researchers first established the science behind the process of 'caloric restriction', as it pertains to human cells, and particularly cancer cells. Prior research has established the value in caloric restriction with respect to retarding cancer cell growth and in enhancing anti-cancer therapies, like chemotherapy. Ongoing caloric restriction with cancer patients is not always feasible, due to the nutritional requirements of some patients.

Researchers compared several methods of inducing caloric restriction, including several pharmaceuticals. They discovered that intermittent fasting was an effective and suitable alternative to these CR mimetic drugs. In addition to IF, they considered other dietary interventions, such as the low carbohydrate/ketogenic diets.

They concluded that intermittent fasting was an excellent method for producing caloric restriction, especially given the fact that the body continued to receive energy from stored energy sources, such as fats, glucose, and triglycerides. With respect to cellular effects, they found:

1. In normal cells, toxicity was reduced and side effects of chemotherapy were reduced
2. In tumor cells, there was an increased sensitivity to chemotherapy treatment and drugs that block cell division
3. Circulation in tumor cells was decreased and tumor size was decreased
4. Enhanced drug delivery effects and tumor die-off

Study #5

Intermittent Fasting in Cardiovascular Disorders— An Overview

This study looked at several contributing areas to cardiovascular disease, and the related benefits of IF. They discovered that the IF diet limited many of the risk factors associated with cardiovascular disease, and the subsequent occurrence of these diseases. By inducing the biochemical transformation of fats, it decreased body mass and reduced blood fats (lipids). It also reduced the concentration of total cholesterol, LDL cholesterol, and triglycerides.

IF also prevented artery hardening by inhibiting the development of atherosclerotic plaque by reducing the concentration of pro-inflammatory markers that contribute to plaque build-up.

IF also inhibited and prevented hypertension. IF causes an increase in the BDNF factor, which results in a lowering of both systolic and diastolic blood pressure by activating the parasympathetic nervous system. This in turn causes acetylcholine to be released by the vagus nerve, resulting in a reduction in heart contractions. The BDNF gene provides instructions for a protein, called the brain-derived neurotrophic factor, that promotes the growth and survival of nerve cells.

Researchers also discovered that IF improved glucose metabolism and increased insulin sensitivity. IF also limits cardiac swelling from cell enlargement.

Study #6

Effects of intermittent fasting on metabolism in men

Metabolic diseases, such as obesity, metabolic syndrome, and type II diabetes have resulted in an increase in the incidence of cardiovascular-related diseases.

This review study confirms what many other studies have previously reported. IF was shown to:

1. Improve blood lipid profiles
2. Decrease inflammatory responses, reflected in serum markers
3. To alter the expression of genes related to inflammation
4. Patient compliance with IF protocols is higher than traditional forms of caloric restriction
5. Reduce oxidative stress
6. Reduce metabolic-related risk factors for cardiovascular disease

Conclusion

While the previous six sample studies contain a good bit of overlapping data and information, when investigating the potential health-related benefits of any treatment protocol, it is always advisable to review multiple research sources in order to compare and verify study results and conclusions. The physiological benefits of IF have been verified through thousands of studies, and appear to have wide-reaching implications for human health and well-being, beyond weight loss and management.

Chapter 8

Prolonged
FASTING

Prolonged fasting, that is fasting for multiple days at a time, is an ancient human practice. Our prehistoric ancestors fasted for prolonged periods, often involuntarily. Availability to food was often unpredictable and uncertain. Food could become unavailable due to natural causes, such as drought, floods, hurricanes, and severe winters. Foodstuff were also more available during certain seasons, especially fresh fruits and vegetables. In prehistoric times, periods without an adequate food supply could last weeks or even months.

Eventually, with the development of agriculture, periods of famine were reduced and ultimately, eliminated. However, some ancient civilizations realized that there were benefits to fasting. Along with the demise of involuntary fasting came the advent of voluntary fasting.

Fasting and the Human Spirit

Throughout history, the practice of fasting was developed independently by different cultures and spiritual traditions. References to fasting are found in the sacred literature of every major world religion. What the ancients discovered was that fasting opens up a window in our consciousness that allows for exceptional human experiences. Our ancestors apparently didn't learn this from other ethnic groups, but instead discovered it on their own through experience.

One way the spiritual aspect of fasting may have been discovered is through asceticism. A sage or mystic may have initiated an abstention from food, purely as a spiritual discipline, only to discover that fasting truly did have spiritual side-effects. Fasting, in this context, is more of a method for pursuing well-being than it is a treatment for disease. This includes the quest for spiritual well-being.

There is an explanation for why some people have exceptional human experiences during prolonged fasts. While rarely discussed or addressed in scientific literature, human beings run off of life energy. We have the power of life active in our bodies while alive. This life energy separates from the physical body at the time of death.

In the East, life energy is not just acknowledged. The traditional medical systems of East Asia and South Asia are predicated upon life energy. In East Asia, Traditional Chinese Medicine refers to life energy as 'chi'. The primary focus of TCM is to prevent disease by uncovering imbalances in the flow of our life energy. Their acupuncture system and their herbal medicine system are both focused on improving the flow of chi, as much or more so than effecting a particular short-term physiological effect.

In India's traditional Ayurvedic medical system, life energy is referred to as 'prana'. Ayurveda takes a balanced approach toward resolving physiological problems, while also working to improve life energy.

Our metabolic processes consume an enormous amount of life energy. When we turn down our metabolism through fasting, we suddenly have a large excess of life energy. Now, this life energy can be utilized by our consciousness to experience aspects of ourselves that are normally unavailable to us, due to our life energy being hard at work in the physical system.

Human potential is vast. We tap only a very small fraction of our mental potential. We also tap only a tiny amount of our spiritual potential. But when our consciousness becomes infused with an abundance of life energy through prolonged fasting, some of this additional mental and spiritual potential begins to manifest. We wake up, so to speak. Our ability to commune with the subtle realms of the super-conscious mind are awakened.

Tapping our spiritual potential through fasting wears no religious or ethnic label. It is a universal, human phenomenon. Many great prophets and sages have reported mystical experiences during episodes of fasting. This is not something that was only true historically. This is as true today as ever. Anyone who wants to experiment with prolonged fasting as a tool for furthering their enlightenment can do so today, as easily as at any other time in history.

Prolonged Fasting Myths

Even though fasting has been widely practiced for ages, many people are taught from an early age that fasting is dangerous. Most of these tales are either mythological or simply ignorance-based. But after myths are repeated continuously, they often become accepted as being true. All of these myths were discredited long ago. However, some of them still persist.

MYTH #1 - Fasting puts you in "starvation mode"

Starvation mode happens when our basal metabolism rate, or BMR, falls to dangerous levels, meaning that our physiological systems have shut down. Research has clearly demonstrated that BMR levels required for metabolic processes and for physical activity are maintained during both prolonged and intermittent fasting.

MYTH #2 - Fasting makes you burn muscle

This myth suggests that when we fast, our bodies immediately turn to muscle as a food and energy source. This is not true. We have evolved to store glucose and fats for energy. The body will not turn to muscle as an energy source, unless fat resources have been depleted. This will not begin to happen until our fat composition drops below 4%. To put this into perspective, lean marathon runners typically carry 8% body fat. Most world-class athletes carry 14% to 20% body fat. People who are considered overweight carry 25% to 31% body fat. If you're obese, you carry over 32% body fat.

MYTH #3 - Fasting causes low blood sugar

Some people are concerned that their blood sugar levels will fall so low that they will become shaky and sweaty. Fortunately, this does not happen when we fast. Our blood glucose levels are closely monitored by our bodies, with several mechanisms working together to maintain these levels within proper ranges. We fast every night as we sleep, and our blood sugar levels are unaffected.

MYTH #4 - Fasting results in overeating

Some studies have shown that on the day when people break a prolonged fast, they tend to eat slightly more on that day; about 20% on average. However, when you factor in the number of calories that were eliminated from the equation, from just one day of fasting, that still means that there is a net deficit in calories totaling 80% of a day's consumption. People who are experienced with fasting, and who fast for multiple days each time, report that their appetite decreases during the fast, and remains low even after refeeding begins.

MYTH #5 - Fasting deprives the body of nutrients

Micronutrients, like vitamins and minerals, are easily available through supplementation. It is a good idea to supplement your diet with micronutrients, whether you're fasting for a prolonged period, or you're practicing intermittent fasting. The longest prolonged fast on record lasted

382 days. A simple multi-vitamin was all that was needed to prevent vitamin deficiency.

We don't need carbohydrates. We do, however, need essential amino acids and essential fatty acids. These cannot be produced from our bodies and must be obtained through diet.

Aminos and fatty acids are expelled in urine and in stool. However, during a fast, our metabolism slows down, and we lose very little. The body can also break down older proteins into their amino acid components, and then recycle them into new proteins. Intermittent fasting protocols will have no issue with a lack of essential aminos and fatty acids. On a longer, prolonged fast, it is always prudent to initiate the fast, and break the fast with meals that are low on carbs and high on proteins and fats.

Longer Periods of Fasting

During longer fasts, results like weight loss and a reduction in insulin levels come fairly quickly and easily. However, anyone who is taking any type of medicine, especially diabetes medicine, should consult with their physician prior to the fast. The physician should monitor all vital signs, especially blood glucose levels. Anyone who initiates a fast longer than a day, should break the fast, if and when they feel ill. Feeling hungry is okay, but not feeling sick. Low blood sugar is expected on a fast, but not at levels so low that they make us feel ill.

The 1968 Extended Fasting Study

An endocrinologist, named Ian Gilliland, organized a fourteen-day, extended fasting research study in 1968 with forty-six patients. He admitted all forty-six subjects into the hospital to ensure compliance and to monitor their progress. During the fast period, his subjects were allowed only water, tea, and coffee. When the fast was completed, he sent his subjects home with instructions for adopting an 800 calorie-per-day diet.

During the fourteen days, his subjects lost an average of 17 pounds. There was also a big drop-off in blood glucose levels, especially beneficial to his three diabetic patients. By the end of the fasting period, they were completely off of insulin.

Another patient who suffered with congestive heart failure, experienced a significant energy boost, and was able to walk and move about without experiencing shortness of breath.

Gilliland asked his patients whether or not they felt the fast was difficult to perform. They replied no. In fact, some said quite the opposite, that it was easy. It left them with feelings of well-being and euphoria. He asked if they felt hungry during the fourteen days. They replied that they encountered hunger after the first day, but that it quickly subsided. Two of his patients asked if they could be readmitted for another fourteen days of fasting. They said they had such good results, that they wanted to achieve even more.

Gilliland sent his patients home with their prescribed 800 calorie-per-day diet, which they were instructed to follow for two years. However, over half of his subjects did not follow these dietary guidelines. It was easier for these patients to fast than it was for them to follow a low-calorie diet.

The Longest Fast

In the 1970's, a Scottish man, weighing in at 456 pounds, began a physician-monitored fast. For 382 days, he lived on non-caloric liquids and dietary supplements, including a daily multivitamin. This fast set the world's record for the longest fast.

After 382 days, he weighed in at 180 pounds. Five years later, he tipped the scales at 196 pounds. His physician who monitored him during the fast reported no harmful health-related effects. During the fast, his blood sugar levels dropped, but remained within the normal range, with no episodes of hypoglycemia.

Extending the Fast

A one-day fast; 24 to 36 hours, is not difficult for most people to do. They will experience some hunger pangs, but it's not a long time; only a day. Extending the fast to two or three days becomes more difficult. Actually, a two-day fast, of 48 to 60 hours is the most difficult fast. The appetite hormone, ghrelin, peaks after a 48-hour fast. After that, it drops off sharply. So, once you're into your third day of fasting, it becomes much easier. For this reason, many fasting experts recommend that, if a person wants to extend a fast into multiple days, it is best to continue the fast for four or five days, or perhaps even longer.

Anyone doing a multiple-day fast, who is new to extended fasting, should consult with a physician prior to the fast, especially if they're taking prescribed medications. For experienced fasters, this may not be necessary, unless the fast extends to seven days or longer. Any fast of this length should be monitored by a physician.

The Beginning

Evidence for the practice of fasting appears in every historic culture and religion. The ancients referred to prolonged fasting periods as times of cleansing, purification, and detoxification. Fasting is mankind's oldest and most time-honored healing tradition.

The ancient Greeks believed strongly in the power of fasting. Plato and Aristotle were both outspoken advocates for fasting. Hippocrates advised that treatment for obesity should include exertion after meals and eating a high-fat diet. He further wrote:

"Sudden death is more common in those who are naturally fat than in the lean. They should, moreover, eat only once a day."

Plutarch agreed. Regarding one of his personal health conditions, he wrote:

"Instead of using medicine, better to fast today."

The Greeks believed that natural remedies could be discovered by observing nature. Since humans, like most mammals, naturally avoid eating when they become sick, they concluded that fasting was a natural remedy for illness. They viewed it as a built-in human instinct.

Fasting has also been a part of the American experience. Benjamin Franklin wrote:

"The best of all medicines is resting and fasting."

Mark Twain wrote:

"A little starvation can really do more for the average sick man than can the best medicines and the best doctors."

Fasting is truly universal, in every sense of the word.

Time to Get Started

Now you've read all about fasting. You know that people have fasted throughout history. You know about fasting methods. You know the science behind fasting. You have much more information than you need to gain an understanding of how fasting will help you. Now it's time to get started. Write down your program, your approach. Decide your start date. This is the end of the Don't Eat That - Intermittent Fasting for Life book, but it is the beginning of your new, improved, and healthier self. And don't forget; we are what we don't eat.